INTERMITTENT FASTING FOR WOMEN OVER 50

The Complete Beginner's Guide to Weight Loss, Increase Energy and Detox your Body

Copyright 2020 - All rights reserved.

This document is geared towards providing exact and reliable information in regards to the topic and issues covered. The publication is sold on the idea that the publisher is not required to render accounting, officially permitted, or otherwise, qualified services. If advice is necessary, legal or professional, a practiced individual in the profession should be ordered.

From a Declaration of Principles which was accepted and approved equally by a Committee of the American Bar Association and a Committee of Publishers and Associations.

In no way is, it legal to reproduce, duplicate, or transmit any part of this document by either electronic means or in printed format. Recording of this publication is strictly prohibited and any storage of this document is not allowed unless with written permission from the publisher. All rights reserved.

The information provided herein is stated to be truthful and consistent, in that any liability, in terms of inattention or otherwise, by any usage or abuse of any policies, processes, or directions contained within is the solitary and utter responsibility of the recipient reader. Under no circumstances will any legal responsibility or blame be held against the publisher for any reparation, damages, or monetary loss due to the information herein, either directly or indirectly.

Respective authors own all copyrights not held by the publisher.

The information herein is offered for informational purposes solely and is universal as so.

The presentation of the information is without a contract or any type of guarantee assurance.

The trademarks that are used are without any consent, and the publication of the trademark is without permission or backing by the trademark owner. All trademarks and brands within this book are for clarifying purposes only and are owned by the owners themselves, not affiliated with this document.

INTRODUCTION

For women who are interested in weight loss, intermittent fasting may seem like a great choice, but many people want to know, should women fast? Is intermittent fasting effective for women? There have been a few key studies about intermittent fasting which can help to shed some light on this interesting new dietary trend.

Intermittent fasting is also known as alternate-day fasting, although there are certainly some variations on this diet. The American Journal of Clinical Nutrition performed a study recently that enrolled 16 obese men and women on a 10-week program. On the fasting days, participants consumed food to 25% of their estimated energy needs. The rest of the time, they received dietary counseling but were not given a specific guideline to follow.

As expected, the participants lost weight due to this experiment, but what researchers really found interesting were some specific changes. The subjects were all still obese after just 10 weeks, but they had shown improvements in cholesterol, LDL-cholesterol, triglycerides, and systolic blood pressure. What made this an interesting find was that most people have to lose more weight than these study participants before seeing the same changes. It was a fascinating find which has spurred a great number of people to try fasting.

Intermittent fasting for women has some beneficial effects. What makes it especially important for women who are trying to lose weight is that women have a much higher fat proportion in their bodies. When trying to lose weight, the body primarily burns through carbohydrate stores within the first 6 hours and then starts to burn fat. Women who are following a healthy diet and exercise plan may be struggling with stubborn fat, but fasting is a realistic solution to this.

This book aims at giving help or guide on intermittent fasting (mainly women) and all these will be explained starting from the history and also give some scientific proof to intermittent fasting, best food and recipes, tip and tricks on how to achieve your (women) desire weight and live a fulfilled life.

TABLE OF CONTENT

INTRODUCTION 4
CHAPTER ONE: INTRODUCTION TO INTERMITTENT FASTING 7
   History of Intermittent Fasting 7
   The Definition of Fasting 12
   Different Types Of Fasting 13
   Intermittent Fasting and Hormone 16
   Intermittent Fasting and Women 17
   When Should You Avoid Intermittent Fasting? 18
   How Do You Know Intermittent Fasting Is Working? 18
   What to Watch Out For 18
   The Science Behind Intermittent Fasting 19
   Advantages of Intermittent Fasting For Women 23
   Stressors And Energy Balance 28
   What To Do Now 29
   Healthy Tips on Intermittent Fasting For Weight Loss 31
CHAPTER TWO: BEST FOOD AND DRINKS FOR INTERMITTENT FASTING 33
   Types of Intermittent Fasting: 34
   Foods For Intermittent Fasting 36
   Healthy Exercise To Support Intermittent Fasting 81
CHAPTER THREE: HEALTHY RECIPES FOR INTERMITTENT FASTING 86
   About The Recipes 86
   Adapting The Recipes To Suit You 86
   HOW TO EAT ON FASTING DAYS...? 115

CHAPTER ONE

INTRODUCTION TO INTERMITTENT FASTING

History of Intermittent Fasting

When it comes to weight loss and what to do to get that trim and sexy figure that you want, there are countless options. You may have heard about exercising, getting your cardio right and dieting. You may have even tried all these methods.

I bet you have not heard anything about Intermittent fasting... right?

Intermittent fasting is simply a way of changing or switching your diet patterns to make sure that you eat during different times in a day.

In ancient Greece, Pythagoras (the sage) was among many who praised the merits of fasting. During the fourteenth century it was practised by St. Catherine of Siena, while the Renaissance doctor Paracelsus named it the ―physician within‖. Indeed, fasting in one form or another is a special tradition and throughout the centuries, devotees have claimed it brings physical and spiritual renewal. During the embryonic cultures, a fast was often required before going to war, or as part of a coming of age ritual. It was used to moderate an angry deity and by native North Americans, as a rite to avoid a disastrous event such as famine.

Fasting has played a vital role in all the world's most famous religions (apart from Zoroastrianism which prohibits it), being related with penitence and other forms of self-control. Judaism has several annual fasting days including Yom Kippur, the Day of

Atonements; in Islam, Muslims fast during the holy month of Ramadan, while Roman Catholics and Eastern orthodoxy observe 40 days fast during Lent, the period when Christ fasted 40 days in the desert.

Women, in particular, seem to have had a tendency for religious fasting, known as ―anorexia mirabilis‖ (miraculous lack of appetite); surviving for periods without nourishment was regarded as a sign of holiness and chastity. Julian of Norwich, an English anchoress, and mystic who lived in the fourteenth century used it as a means of communicating with Christ.

In other belief systems, the gods were thought to reveal their divine teaching in dreams and visions only after a fast by the temple priests.

Also another reason for this can be seen from the political aspect, fasting has also long been used as a gesture of political protest, the classic example being the Suffragettes and Mahatma Gandhi who undertook 17 fasts during the struggle for Indian independence: his longest fast lasted 21 days. But the practice has also had its dark side, having been exploited by exhibitionists and fraudsters, and foisted on the naive. Take ―Doctor‖ Linda Burfield Hazzard, from Minnesota, thought to have caused the death of over 40 patients whom she put on strict fasts, before being convicted of manslaughter in 1912. She died from her fasting regime in 1938. Then there were the Victorian ―fasting girls‖ who claimed to be able to survive indefinitely without food; one of them, Sarah Jacobs, was allowed to starve to death aged 12 as doctors tested her claims in hospital. Therapeutic fasting in which fasting is used to either treat or prevent ill health, with medical supervision became popular in the 19th century as part of the ―Natural Hygiene Movement‖ in the US. Doctor Herbert Shelton was one revered pioneer, opening ―Doctor Shelton's Health school‖ in San Antonio, Texas, in 1928. He claimed to have helped 40,000 patients recover their health with water fast.

In the UK, too, fasting became part of the ―Nature Cure‖, an approach which also stressed the importance of exercise, diet, sunshine, fresh air and ―positive thinking‖. ―Fasting was at its most popular here in the 1920s,‖ according to Tom Greenfield, a naturopath who runs a clinic in Canterbury. ―The first Nature Cure clinic to offer fasting opened in Edinburgh and I still have one or two patients who fasted there many decades ago.‖ Other clinics which offered therapeutic fasting included the legendary Tyringham Hall in Buckinghamshire, now closed, and Champneys in Tring, Hertfordshire, in those days a naturopathic Centre, now a destination spa.

Fasting was used to treat heart disease, high blood pressure, obesity, digestive problems, allergies, headaches pretty much everything. Fasts were individually tailored and could be anything from a day or two to three months, for obese patients. The clinics would take a full case history to see if people were suitable and they would be closely monitored.

Eventually, scientific medicine became dominant as better drugs were developed: fasting and the ―Nature Cure‖ fell out of favour in Britain. By contrast, in Germany where fasting was pioneered by Dr. Otto Buchinger, therapeutic fasting is still popular and offered at various centers. Many German hospitals now run fasting weeks, funded by health insurance programs, to help manage obesity, while fasting holidays at centers and spas throughout Europe, including Hungary, the Czech Republic, and Austria, are growing in popularity. ―In Germany fasting is part of the naturheilkunde (natural health practice),‖ says Greenfield. ―It has remained popular because it became integrated into medical practice so patients could be referred for a fast by their doctors.‖

More recently, interest in fasting has come back to limelight in the UK, with millions trying intermittent fasting such as the 5:2 diets, or on modified fasts where only certain foods or juices are taken for a period. Greenfield welcomes the renewed interest and says: ―If people can do a one day fast for a minimum of twice a year – maybe one in spring and one in the autumn and setting aside a day they can rest, when they just drink water – this will help mitigate the toxic effects of daily living.‖

I will digress a bit to show the problems of obesity which can be helped thanks to fasting. And how to go about these problems.

Over the past few years, obesity has ceased or stopped being an exclusively aesthetic problem and has crossed the line to become a health and healthcare issue, by turning into a genuine worldwide epidemic requiring enormous human, technical, and economic resources to fight. In spite of the deployment of massive preventives and therapeutic arsenals by political, medical, scientific authorities, obesity has, far from stopping, multiplied dangerously. Its increment in society has reached such a point that experts have started to call it ―globesity‖, a sub-species of fatness globalization, irrespective of a country's status as developed or underdeveloped. Recent epidemiological studies show that a high percentage of people have some kind of pathology associated with excess weight, reaching figures exceeding 300 million all over the world.

The alarm bells sound even louder when data on child and youth obesity is examined. These nutritional disorders entail some of the disorders associated with excess weight, some of them chronic, such as type diabetes, heart diseases, high blood pressure and even different types of cancer.

The obesity disorder has also considerably affected children, as already mentioned, since the number of obese people has multiplied or increased in the studies carried out in developed countries such as the United States and some in Europe, mainly due to a change in eating habits, above all in the consumption of fat and a considerable reduction in physical activity.

About anti-obesity treatments, these continue to produce unsatisfactory results which are often due to mistaken strategies and the improper use of the therapeutic resources available and applied. According to estimations of the World Health Organization (WHO), the cause of death of 41 million of the 64 million people who died in 2015 wer chronic diseases. Pathologies associated with obesity, such as diabetes, hypertension, cardiovascular diseases or the metabolic syndrome will monopolize 80% of healthcare expenditures in the next ten years. For all these reasons, and given the extremely high economic costs meant for Public Health Systems at its roots to be able to fight or address this in its branches. It seems obligatory to deploy a worldwide inter- and multi-disciplinary structure of professionals helping to fight this disease of epidemic proportions spread all over the planet: a system made up of specialists in different areas, from primary healthcare doctors, endocrinologists, nutritionists, psychologists, physical education teachers or working politicians.

Obesity is a chronic problem of individual and public health which affects a large number of people all over the world. Stopping its invasion and succeeding in maintaining healthy lifestyles to revert this situation is the responsibility of all social agents involved.

Going back to fasting, the majority of people fast for a religious purpose. The scientific reason behind fasting is Insulin hormone and few other hormones that work well in the fasted state. Insulin is a fat deposit hormone. Needless spike of insulin is not wanted. Insulin spike will cause fat deposit around waist visceral fat, which is the most difficult to burn once built. Thousands of diabetic and obese patient or people have adapted to Intermittent Fasting of eating one meal a day. Apart from controlling blood sugar, eating just one meal a day brings several more benefits - reducing waist size, increasing muscle through increased HGH hormone assuming the single meal is not void of protein, reduced blood pressure, improved lipid profile through lower LDL/Triglycerides and higher HDL, reduced CRP or inflammation, sound sleep, alert brain, increased activity at work and in physical exercises and cure of other ailments such as headache, body ache, and so on.

In some religions and spiritualities, fasting is a way to cleanse and purify the body and is considered an act of sacrifice. Fasting can also be used to reduce or lose weight in cases of morbid obesity. Some individuals use fasting as a means to detoxify their body. Other times, medical testing or surgery may be compulsory in the period of fasting before the procedure. I will like to define fasting.

The Definition of Fasting

What makes fasting seem so novel is that, with all the diet advice out there, the easiest might be to simply not eat. Of course, fasting is not the same as starving yourself, which is what the majority think when they hear —fasting.‖ And yet, fasting is not a diet, either. The literal definition of fasting is to refrain from food and drink from a specific period it's been in existence for decades or years, as spiritual fasting is a part of many religions. But in this context, I prefer defining fasting as —an act of change in eating patterns

In place of three square meals a day or a handful of smaller meals throughout the day, you will have a specific schedule of time when you are eating, whether it is a few hours a day or certain days of the week. During that time, you can eat whatever you want. Of course, I say that within reason. If you are eating processed foods and potato chips, it is unlikely you will reap the benefits of fasting. If that is you, I encourage you to examine your diet before trying a fast. But if you practice fasting and stick to a mostly whole food diet, rich in fruits, veggies, lean proteins, healthy fats and raw dairy, you will see changes and for those occasional splurges on chocolate or cheese would not have as big of an impact as they might if you were on a calorie-restrictive diet. The beauty of fasting is that there is no one ―right‖ way to do it. In fact, there are several types that are popular. And this I will like to put forward in their types.

Different Types Of Fasting

1. Intermittent Fasting

This type of fasting is also known as cyclic fasting. Intermittent fasting is a catch-all phrase for eating (and not eating) intermittently. In fact, almost all of the fasting methods below are types of intermittent fasting! Typical intermittent fast times range from 14 to 18 hours. The longest period any one of these plans would require you to abstain from solid food would be about 32–36 hours.

2. Time-Restricted Eating

If you practice time-restricted eating, you will abstain from food for anywhere between 12– 16 hours. During your eating window, you can eat as much of your favorite healthy foods as you'd like. This is one of the most common methods of fasting. Time-restricted eating is pretty simple to implement. If you finish dinner at 7 p.m., for instance, you will not eat anything again until at least 7 a.m. If you wanted to take it further, you'd extend the no-eating time until about 11 a.m. or 12 p.m. Because you are sleeping for a large chunk of the ―no eating‖ time, this is a good way to introduce fasting into your lifestyle and experiment without any major changes.

This is another name for time-restricted eating, here you will fast for 16 hours a day and then eat the other eight.

3. Alternate Day Fasting

Another type of intermittent fasting, alternate day fasting has you severely restricting the number of calories you eat during fasting days, then eating to your stomach's content on non-fasting days. Food is not completely off the table, but you will stick to about 25 percent of your normal caloric intake. Someone eating 2,000 calories would cut back to 500, for example. Alternate-day fasting is not necessarily a long-term plan, because it can become difficult to stick to, but it can be helpful to get a healthy habit in motion.

4. Daniel's Fasting

This is very similar to alternate day fasting except here you eat normally for five days of the week. On the other two, calories are restricted to about 500–600 calories a day. Another type of fasting. Here, you will stick to fruits and veggies during the day and then eat a well-rounded, larger meal in the day. This is a type of spiritual fasting. Based off of Daniel's experiences in the Bible's Book of Daniel, the Daniel Fast is a partial fast where vegetables, fruits and other healthy whole foods are featured prominently, but meat, dairy, grains (unless they're sprouted ancient grains) and drinks like coffee, alcohol, and juice are avoided.

Most people follow this fast for 21 days in order to experience a spiritual breakthrough, have more time to reflect on their relationship with God or just to feel closer to what Daniel would have experienced in his time.

Fasting is an ancient method of healing that has been practiced for thousands of years. In modern Western culture, we have lost touch with these and other ancient mind-body practices, but fasting is making a comeback due to its health benefits.

You might have likely come across intermittent fasting and the scientifically-backed 3 (three) days fast to reset your immune system.

Fasting may indeed have some benefits, and intermittent fasting can be beneficial for weight loss, but as with all things diet and health-related, there is never a one size fits all panacea. Women especially may want to more carefully consider using fasting as a health tool.

First off: what is fasting? You probably know fasting is willingly withholding food for a determined period. Used therapeutically, this is typically one to three days, but mileage varies. Intermittent fasting (IF) is a little different and involves a brief fast of 12-16 hours. Most of us are fasting overnight between dinner and breakfast anyway, but intermittent fasting (IF) is a little more calculated. Some people eat only during an 8 (eight) hours window during the day; some take a whole 24 fast, and others simply fast for a specific window overnight. It gets way detailed when you go down the intermittent fasting.

This intermittent fasting has some benefits. Which I will highlight below, fasting for 12 + hours each day has promising health benefits. It might help extend your life due to cellular and hormonal benefits. It may also regulate blood glucose levels, control blood lipids, maintain lean mass, and assists with weight loss. It can improve cell turnover, reduce inflammation, and assist with appetite regulation. It could also slow the ageing process: During the fasting phase, cells die and stem cells are activated, which starts a regeneration process and gives rise to new, younger cells.

My special idea is when you give your body a good 12+ hour chunk of time with no food; especially overnight, it is better able to focus on detoxification and repair. Also, when you are fasting, your body relies on stored glycogen for fuel, and when that's exhausted, it uses the only next best of energy: stored fat. You want this if your goal is to lose weight and burn fat.

Notwithstanding, Intermittent fasting may not be the holy grail for everyone. It can be seen from another perspective which is entirely different from the religious, political and any other claims mention at the initial stage.

Intermittent Fasting and Hormone

It should be made clear that our bodies want us to make babies and continue to populate the earth. Women especially have delicate endocrine systems that basically drive us to prevent starvation and excessive stress so we can protect a developing fetus. So you can blame cravings and excessive appetite on biology in many cases, but the roots are in unbalanced hormones. If the female body senses starvation or stress, hunger hormones increase to drive you to chow down.

Intermittent fasting can spur this response in some women. Our hunger hormones, ghrelin and leptin, tell us when to eat and when we are full. In fact, Women are more susceptible to ramped up ghrelin production after fasting, as we discussed above. This can cause binge eating in response to fasting and may exacerbate disordered eating behavior. Fasting or intermittent fasting can affect thyroid function and fertility in some women, especially if it is not done properly, done too often, or the woman already has weak adrenals or hormone imbalance.

In fact, studies on rats by researchers show that after two weeks of intermittent fasting, female rats stopped having menstrual cycles and their ovaries shrunk. They also experienced more insomnia than their male counterparts (though the male rats did experience lower testosterone production). Human bodies may not perform like rats obviously, but there is not yet much research on intermittent fasting and benefits for women, I will explain what is known below.

Intermittent Fasting and Women

This saying is rampant, telling women not to involve themselves in intermittent fasting. This often steered women away from intermittent fasting, but I do think it has benefits. The key here is that, knowing if intermittent fasting is right for you and how to intermittent fasting properly for your body.

With several experiences, intermittent fasting for 14-16 hours works very well for obese women; women who have more than 30 pounds to lose; and women with high blood sugar and high lipids. Who should not involve in intermittent fasting: If you have a history of eating disorders, you have hypoglycemia, you have adrenal fatigue or hypothyroidism that is not yet dialed in, or you are underweight, you may want to think twice. Not all women who are pregnant, want to become pregnant, or who have had trouble conceiving should steer clear of intermittent fasting. If you are a woman who is regular weight for your height, or you have 10 or so pounds to lose, the best way to intermittent fasting is a few non-consecutive days weekly. This means you do not need to involve yourself in intermittent fasting every day, only two or three days a week let's say. You'd fast for 12-16 hours (aim for 14-16), which is not that difficult. It means you stop eating after dinner at 7 pm and then do not eat anything again until 7 am earliest the following morning. You can have water, coffee, or tea, but no milk or sweeteners in these liquids and nothing else.

For women, if you are a woman and you have more than 30 pounds to lose, you can try Intermittent fasting often, 5-7 days a week even. You also have the option of fasting one full 24 hours a week. There are many different options; you just need to see what works for your body.

When Should You Avoid Intermittent Fasting?

Intermittent fasting isn't a good fit for everyone. You shouldn't consider intermittent fasting if you are:

- Pregnant
- Nursing
- Under chronic stress
- Have a previous history of disordered eating, such as bulimia or anorexia
- Struggle with sleep disorders, or have difficulty sleeping

How Do You Know Intermittent Fasting Is Working?

If intermittent fasting is working for you, you will notice that your weight has reduced or you lose weight (if that is your aim), improved blood sugar balance (works best if you can monitor this with a glucometer), energy boost, good sleep. You feel good.

What to Watch Out For

If you are trying intermittent fasting you notice any of the following, you may need to make adjustments: you are starving and shaky. Intermittent fasting spurs binge behavior you notice a change in your menstrual cycle you have missed periods you are otherwise cranky or irritable

If you were going for a full 16 hours, try just 12. If you were doing it every day, try only 2-3 days a week. Make some adjustments and revisit. If it is still not working, you can add in some adaptogenic herbs to support your endocrine system.

Though, not everyone needs intermittent fasting. But I do recommend at least a 10 hour fast overnight to gives your body a chance to repair itself while you sleep. It cannot focus on it is night duties when you have a belly full of food to digest. That is a reason people do not sleep well when they eat a big meal and go to bed. If you have tired adrenals or hypoglycemia, or you cannot sleep through the night, you may need a small before bed snack to support blood sugar, and that is a sign that you should work on regulating blood sugar and nourishing your hormones before you can successfully Although advocates boast the euphoric-like benefits they experience from restricted eating times, very little if anything is discussed in current research about the impacts of intermittent fasting on women's health particularly hormones, the female brain, energy and long-term benefits and/or consequences.

Many women ask this questions:

i. Is intermittent fasting bad for women?

ii. What if anything happens to women's hormones when they intermittent fast?

iii. And how, if at all, are women different, from men, when it comes to the benefits from intermittent fasting?

The Science Behind Intermittent Fasting

Hormones play a large role in our body. Each hormone has its function and performance. Our growth hormone is the one responsible for helping us burn fat. When we fast, our growth hormone starts working overtime burning fat at a much faster rate. Fasting also keeps our insulin levels down so we're burning the fat instead of storing it in our body.

In order for our hormones to burn fat, they need fat burning enzymes to do their part as well. Adipose tissue HSL and Muscle tissue LPL are the two most important fat burning enzymes. HSL helps the body release fat and turn it into energy and muscles while LPL helps the cells in our muscles store the fat so it can be burnt as fuel. When working together, these enzymes will help the hormones burn fat twice as fast. Intermittent fasting allows these hormones and enzymes to burn the fat quickly on the day you fast.

Fasting is a great way to keep the body and mind healthy and clean. Many people that practice intermittent fasting regularly claim they've learned a lot about their eating habits as well. The reason is that they have a lot of time to think about food and which foods they're craving on their fasting days. The level of adrenaline your body produces is also increased during short-term fasting, which puts your body's ability to burn fat into overdrive and work twice as hard. Combine this with your increased metabolism and you can see how losing weight would be so common with intermittent fasting.

Many diet and exercise trends have origins in legitimate science, though the facts tend to get distorted by the time they achieve mainstream popularity. Benefits are exaggerated. Risks are downplayed. Science takes a back seat to marketing.

So popular, in fact, that it is quickly moving into fad territory, suggests Pilon. And when something becomes a fad intensely popular but only for a short period several problems typically ensue. For one, he says, many doctors and nutrition experts are prone to dismissing fads out of hand. So their patients and clients, while shielded from the ridiculous claims of overzealous dieting evangelists, may also lose out on the legitimate benefits of fasting done right.

Another concern is that promoters of intermittent fasting will, perhaps unintentionally, encourage extreme behaviour, such as bingeing. The implication being that if you fast two days a week, you can devour as much junk as your gullet can swallow during the remaining five days.

Not so, say more moderate proponents of fasting. Their take on intermittent fasting: eat sensibly most of the time, eat nothing for an extended period every now and then, indulge only on occasion (perhaps once a week, say, on a designated —cheat day‖). There is research, they claim, to back up the health benefits of sensibly incorporating fasting into your lifestyle.

There is indeed a large body of research to support the health benefits of fasting, though most of it has been conducted on animals, not humans. Still, the results have been promising. Fasting has been shown to improve biomarkers of disease, reduce oxidative stress and preserve learning and memory functioning, according to Mark Mattson, senior investigator for the National Institute on Aging, part of the US National Institutes of Health. Mattson has investigated the health benefits of intermittent fasting on the cardiovascular system and brain in rodents, and has called for —well-controlled human studies‖ in people —across a range of body mass indexes.

There are several theories about why fasting provides physiological benefits, says Mattson. —The one that we've studied a lot, and designed experiments to test, is the hypothesis that during the fasting period, cells are under a mild stress,‖ he says. —And they respond to the stress adaptively by enhancing their ability to cope with stress and, maybe, to resist disease.‖

Though the word —stress‖ is often used in a negative sense, taxing the body and mind has benefits. Consider vigorous exercise, which stresses, in particular, muscles and the cardiovascular system. As long as you give your body time to recover, it will grow stronger.

—There is considerable similarity between how cells respond to the stress of exercise and how cells respond to intermittent fasting,‖ says Mattson.

Mattson has contributed to several other studies on intermittent fasting and caloric restriction. In one, overweight adults with moderate asthma consumed only 20% of their normal calorie intake on alternate days. Participants who adhered to the diet lost 8% of their initial body weight over eight weeks. They also saw a decrease in markers of oxidative stress and inflammation, and improvement of asthma-related symptoms and several quality-of-life indicators.

In another study, Mattson and colleagues explored the effects of intermittent and continuous energy restriction on weight loss and various biomarkers (for conditions including breast cancer, diabetes and cardiovascular disease) among young overweight woman. They found that intermittent restriction was as effective as continuous restriction for improving weight loss, insulin sensitivity and other health biomarkers.

Mattson has also researched the protective benefits of fasting to neurons. If you don't eat for 10–16 hours, your body will go to its fat stores for energy, and fatty acids called ketones will be released into the bloodstream. This has been shown to protect memory and learning functionality, says Mattson, as well as slow disease processes in the brain.

But perhaps it isn't so much the fasting that produces health benefits, per se, as the resulting overall reduction in calorie intake (if, that is, you don't overeat on nonfasting days, which could create a caloric surplus instead of a deficit).

—Caloric restriction, undernutrition without malnutrition, is the only experimental approach consistently shown to prolong survival in animal models,‖ Freedland and colleagues stated in a study on the effects of intermittent fasting on prostate cancer growth in mice. In the study, mice fasted twice a week for 24 hours, but were otherwise permitted to eat at liberty. During nonfasting days, the mice overate. Overall, they did not lose weight, counteracting whatever benefits they might have seen from fasting. Intermittent fasting with compensatory overeating —did not improve mouse survival nor did it delay prostrate tumor growth,‖ the study concluded.

To improve health, the goal should be to lose weight by reducing the total amount of calories consumed, suggests Freedland, rather than focusing on when those calories are consumed. —If you don't eat two days a week, and limit what you eat the other five days, you will lose weight. It's one approach to losing weight,‖ he says. —I'm not sure it works any better than cutting down slightly seven days a week.

Advantages of Intermittent Fasting For Women

I. If You Have Body Fat to Lose or Want to Spike Your Metabolism, Intermittent Fasting May Help You See results.

For those desiring healthy body fat or weight loss, intermittent fasting can help spark your metabolism and body's ability to burn fat at least in the short term. Intermittent fasting has been shown to reduce body fat, while preserving lean muscle mass, in both men and women, as it boosts —human growth factor‖ (i.e. lean muscle mass), in turn raising metabolism (your body has more muscle to —burn‖ or feed). However, take these claims with a grain of salt. Men (compared to women) still tend to experience —greater results‖ with intermittent fasting.

A. study from cardiologists at the Intermountain Medical Center revealed that human growth factor levels were elevated by 2000 percent in men and ―only‖ 1300 percent in women (Intermountain Medical Center, 2011). In other words: All the marketing claims that boast, ―lose body fat‖ with fasting may be talking more to men. Nevertheless, many women with

extra body fat may see benefits initially.

II. Intermittent Fast Can Be A Positive Stress Not All Stress Is Bad.

We call positive stress ―eustress‖ and a little bit does a body good. Just like exercise stress helps you build a fitter body, ―hard times‖ make you stronger and winter cold helps us appreciate summer heat, intermittent fasting periods of not eating can also be a positive ―stressor‖ for actually allowing your body to take a break from eating, followed by a period of nourishment and replenishment.

In fact, for some, intermittent fasting is actually a positive stressor for promoting a state of ―rest and digest‖ a break from feeding may feel uncomfortable at first, but as the body adapts, your body actually has been an opportunity to take advantage of a recovery (from eating) window, wherein it can fully absorb and digest the foods you have eaten.

III. You May Conquer Cravings

Intermittent fasting and fasting has shown proven benefits for regulating blood sugar and taming cravings (particularly for things your imbalanced blood sugar craves like sugar, refined foods and caffeine).

(Arnason et al, 2017). A review of studies (Carlson et al, 20017) of individuals who fasted, versus those who just restricted calories, found fasting individuals experienced ―greater‖ insulin sensitivity improvements (20-30% change), and one more study found that intermittent fasting did not negatively affect Ghrelin levels (hunger hormone) meaning it did not make people —hungrier‖ simply because they did not eat for a window of time (Alzoghaibi et al, 2014).

IV. Intermittent Fasting Cuts Diabetes And Heart Disease Risks

Intermittent fasting with water might just bring down your heart disease risks and chances of developing diabetes. The research was conducted in an area where up to 65% of the population are Mormons who, in observance of their faith, fast one day every month.

Interesting that heart disease rates are consistently lowest in this area. Until recently, many experts attributed this to the fact the Mormon Church discourages smoking by members. However, even though the number of smokers has decreased across the U.S., Utah continues to have a heart disease rate that is lower than the rest.

In earlier work, the same research team found that subjects who answered "yes" when asked whether they fasted had less heart disease. The latest study sought to reproduce and take these earlier results further, to see if this might be the reason for the lower heart disease risk.

In an accompanying study, the researchers examined blood markers for heart risks in those who hadn't fasted over the last 12 hours. The markers were reviewed when the subjects fasted and also monitored during a normal day of eating. The fasts were water only, though participants were allowed to take medication.

During the fast, the levels of good cholesterol (HDL) rose, as did LDL (bad) cholesterol and total cholesterol numbers – not favorable to be sure, but the researchers believe the rise may be temporary. But, those fasting also had reductions in dangerous blood fats known as triglycerides, as well as blood sugar levels. When you fast, the body tries to preserve its cells and tissue, using fats instead of sugars for fuel.

V. Intermittent Fasting for Women Can Help You Simplify Food:

Food is not complicated. However, the diet, health and weight loss industry often makes it out to be. You were born with a natural intuition that tells you when you're hungry, full and what (real‿) foods your body needs—a balance of proteins (amino acids), healthy fats (fatty acids) and ―sugars‖ (carbohydrates with glucose), and a variety of micro-nutrients (vitamins and minerals) available in all sorts of foods. Somewhere along the way, we got confused and stopped learning how to listen to our body and trust our body. Intermittent fasting can help take unnecessary time spent calorie counting, dreaming about your next meal or feeling like you have to eat based on a 5-6 meal/ day schedule versus, eating and nourishing your body with abundance of real whole foods during a chunk of time in the day then going on with your life. Not over thinking food.

Intermittent fasting has shown proven benefits for unhealthy individuals such as those with obesity, overweight, diabetes and insulin sensitivity at least in the short term. However, even for these individuals once improved health markers are attained, normalized eating habits (regular eating) and peace with food may prove most beneficial for all women in the long run.

Also to crown it all, perhaps most importantly, if you are already under a significant amount of stress or see intermittent fasting with the ―diet mentality,‖ then intermittent fasting may also stress your body out more. Face it, stress is inevitable and we already face a fair amount of stress in a given week. Women's bodies walk a more delicate line (at least compared to men), and the addition of stress turned up a notch without care to address that stress can throw your hormones and body —balance‖ over the edge.

Sure, we do our best to be healthy and battle these stressors, but if we do not carefully pay attention to managing and recovering from stress in our daily lives, another body stressor like intermittent fasting can throw more fuel to the fire sending your body (cortisol and other hormones included) into the —overboard‖ zone.

For some, not eating is the last thing their body desires when it already has enough stress to face, and as it is forced to work even harder (to sustain your energy levels), hormone imbalances, mood imbalances, disordered eating habits and the diet mentality can happen more.

Coming from a girl who's walked the walk and talked the talk (yours truly) and tried every single dieting or eating philosophy under the sun (intermittent fasting included), if there's one thing I have learned about intermittent fasting for women is that: unless you are in a place (in your head and your health) to truly listen to your body, and nourish it completely (instead of treat it like an object or project to manipulate, force or confirm), intermittent fasting is not for you.

Well, so women's hormonal balance is particularly sensitive to how much, how often, and what we eat. But how do our bodies —know‖ when food is scarce? For many years, scientists believed that it was a woman's body fat percentage that regulated her reproductive system. The idea was that if a woman fat reserve dipped below a certain percentage (somewhere around 11 percent might be a reasonable guess), hormones would get messed up and your period would stop. Boom: no risk of pregnancy.

This makes a lot of sense. If there is not much to eat, you'll lose body fat over time. But the situation is actually more complicated than that. After all, food availability can change quickly. And as you probably know if you have ever tried to lose weight your body fat often takes a while to drop, even if you are eating fewer calories.

Meanwhile, women who are not lean can also stop ovulating and lose their periods. That is why scientists have come to suspect that overall energy balance may be more important to this process than body fat percentage.

Stressors And Energy Balance

Specifically, negative energy balance in women may be to blame for the hormonal domino effect we've been talking about. And it's not just about how much food you eat. Negative energy balances can result from: too little food, poor nutrition, too much exercise, too much stress, illness, infection, chronic inflammation, too little rest and recovery.

Heck, we can even use up energy reserves by trying to keep warm. Any combination of these stressors could be enough to put you into negative energy balance and stop ovulation: training for a marathon and nursing flu; too many days in a row at the gym and not enough fruits and vegetables; intermittent fasting and busting your butt to pay the mortgage.

Psychological stress can absolutely play a role in damaging our hormonal equilibrium.

Our bodies cannot tell the difference between a real threat and something imaginary generated by our thoughts and feelings.

The stress hormone cortisol inhibits our friend GnRH and suppresses the ovaries' production of estrogen and progesterone. Meanwhile, progesterone is converted to cortisol during stress, so more cortisol means less progesterone. This leads to estrogen dominance in the HPG axis. You could be hovering at 30 percent fat. But if your energy balance is negative for a long enough time, especially if you are stressed, reproduction stops.

What To Do Now

Based on what we know intermittent fasting probably affects reproductive health if the body sees it as a significant stressor. Anything that affects your reproductive health affects your overall health and fitness. Even if you do not plan to have kids. But intermittent fasting protocols vary, with some being much more extreme than others. And factors such as your age, your nutritional status, the length of time you fast, and the other stresses in your life including exercise are also likely relevant.

Considering how much remains unclear, I would suggest a conservative approach. If you want to try IF, begin with a gentle protocol, and pay attention to how things are going.

Stop intermittent fasting if your menstrual cycle stops or becomes irregular, you have problems falling asleep or staying asleep, your hair falls out, you start to develop dry skin or acne, you are noticing you do not recover from workouts as easily, your injuries are slow to heal, or you get every bug going around, your tolerance to stress decreases, your moods start swinging, your heart starts going pitter-patter in a weird way, your interest in romance fizzles (and your lady parts stop appreciating it when it happens), your digestion system functions slowly, you always seem to feel cold

Fasting is not for everyone the truth is, some women should not even bother experimenting. Do not try intermittent fasting if you are pregnant, you have a history of disordered eating, you are chronically stressed, you do not sleep well, you are not familiar with diet and exercise. Pregnant women have extra energy needs.

So if you are starting a family, fasting is not a good idea. As said earlier, if you are under chronic stress or if you are not sleeping well. Your body needs nurturing, not additional stress. And if you have struggled with disordered eating in the past, you probably recognize that a fasting protocol could lead you down a path that might create further problems for you. Instead of engaging in intermittent fasting You can achieve similar benefits in other ways.

If you are used to diet and exercise, intermittent fasting might look like a magic bullet for weight loss. But you'd be a lot smarter to address any nutritional deficiencies before you start experimenting with fasts. Ensure you are starting from a solid nutritional foundation first.

What to do if fasting is not for you, how can you get in shape and lose weight if intermittent fasting is not a good option for you. It is simple, really. Learn the essentials of good nutrition. It is by far the best thing you can do for your health and fitness. Cook and eat whole foods. Exercise regularly. Stay consistent. And if you'd like some help to do all of that, hire a coach. Sure, intermittent fasting may be popular. And maybe your brother or your boyfriend or your husband or even your dad finds it an excellent aid to fitness and health. But women are different than men and our bodies have different needs. Observe your body. And do what works best for you.

Healthy Tips on Intermittent Fasting For Weight Loss

1. Don't Make Your Fast Too Long Or Too Short

An ideal fast length for weight-loss and health benefits is between 16 and 24 hours depending on age, experience and exact goals. Any less than this won't really give you the results you want (remember you are already fasting for 10-12 hours overnight) and any longer than this is simply unnecessary and can be harder to adapt to.

2. Increase Your Water Intake When Fasting

Intermittent fasting will also help to cleanse your system and let your body work more efficiently. In order to help with this process, you should increase your water intake. The best way to do this is have a glass/bottle of water with you at all times so that you can sip regularly.

3. BreakYour Fast With A Healthy Meal

The first thing you eat after a fast should be a healthy meal. Apart from the obvious benefits of eating healthy food, this also leaves less space for eating junk. Given that you might only have 8 hours to eat your daily food, filling up on the good stuff first is always a good option.

4. Time Your Food Around Your Workouts

It goes without saying that working out should be part of any healthy eating plan. The centrepiece of your training efforts should be weight-training or bodyweight training. Try to eat most of your food in the period immediately after your workout. In this way, your body will be more likely to use these calories to rebuild and repair rather than be stocked as fat.

5. Don't Sweat The Details

One of the real benefits of intermittent fasting is that it is not necessary to count calories or grams of macronutrients. This can be a pain and makes diets difficult to stick to. Follow principles and the details will take care of themselves.

CHAPTER TWO

BEST FOOD AND DRINKS FOR INTERMITTENT FASTING

It is important to realize that the key is actually nutrition and finding an approach that works for you long-term. This is where an intermittent fasting diet is a particularly interesting option when compared to other dietary approaches.

So does an intermittent fasting diet work when compared to other diets? The answer here is a resounding yes. For example, using a 16 hour fast will keep your body burning fat for most of every day! And getting all of your calories during a relatively small eating window stops your body from going into starvation mode and desperately hanging onto body-fat. Compared to a normal reduced calorie diet, this is a huge difference. While any reduced calorie approach will initially lead to fat-loss, your body is an efficient machine and will compensate by slowing down your metabolism (the exact opposite of what you want) and holding onto body fat.

Is Intermittent Fasting Diet Restrictive? Any diet, by its very nature, involves making better food choices. If someone tries to sell you on the pancake diet, run a mile! Eating rubbish can never be a good choice. However, most diets will have you try to eat clean all the time. This is very hard to do and is directly linked to finding yourself eating 12 doughnuts in one sitting after a couple of weeks of deprivation! Intermittent fasting also involves healthy food choices, but it does give you more wiggle room. It is difficult to eat too much junk in a small eating window after you have already had your healthy food. It does let you eat enough to stop you falling off the wagon, however.

Types of Intermittent Fasting:

Intermittent fasting comes in various forms and each may have a specific set of unique benefits. Each form of intermittent fasting has variations in the fasting-to-eating ratio. The benefits and effectiveness of these different protocols may differ on an individual basis and it is important to determine which one is best for you.

Factors that may influence which one to choose include health goals, daily schedule/routine, and current health status. The most common types of IF are alternate day fasting, time-restricted feeding, and modified fasting.

1. Alternate Day Fasting:

This approach involves alternating days of absolutely no calories (from food or beverage) with days of free feeding and eating whatever you want.

This plan has been shown to help with weight loss, improve blood cholesterol and triglyceride (fat) levels, and improve markers for inflammation in the blood.

The main downfall with this form of intermittent fasting is that it is the most difficult to stick with because of the reported hunger during fasting days.

2. Modified Fasting - 5:2 Diet

Modified fasting is a protocol with programmed fasting days, but the fasting days do allow for some food intake. Generally, 20-25% of normal calories are allowed to be consumed on fasting days; so if you normally consume 2000 calories on regular eating days, you would be allowed 400-500 calories on fasting days. The 5:2 part of this diet refers to the ratio of non-fasting to fasting days. Soon this regimen you would eat normally for 5 consecutive days, then fast or restrict calories to 20-25% for 2 consecutive days.

This protocol is great for weight loss, body composition, and may also benefit the regulation of blood sugar, lipids, and inflammation. Studies have shown the 5:2 protocol to be effective for weight loss, improve/lower inflammation markers in the blood (3), and show signs of trending improvements in insulin resistance. In animal studies, this modified fasting 5:2 diet resulted in decreased fat, decreased hunger hormones (leptin), and increased levels of a protein responsible for improvements in fat burning and blood sugar regulation (adiponectin).

The modified 5:2 fasting protocol is easy to follow and has a small number of negative side effects which included hunger, low energy, and some irritability when beginning the program. Contrary to this, however, studies have also noted improvements such as reduced tension, less anger, less fatigue, improvements in self-confidence, and a more positive mood.

3. Time-Restricted Feeding:

If you know anyone that has said they are doing intermittent fasting, odds are it is in the form of time-restricted feeding. This is a type of intermittent fasting that is used daily and it involves only consuming calories during a small portion of the day and fasting for the remainder. Daily fasting intervals in time-restricted feeding may range from 12-20 hours, with the most common method being 16/8 (fasting for 16 hours, consuming calories for 8). For this protocol, the time of day is not important as long as you are fasting for a consecutive period of time and only eating in your allowed time period. For example, on a 16/8 time-restricted feeding program one person may eat their first meal at 7AM and last meal at 3 PM (fast from 3PM-7AM), while another person may eat their first meal at 1 PM and last meal at 9 PM (fast from 9PM-1PM). This protocol is meant to be performed every day over long periods of time and is very flexible as long as you are staying within the fasting/eating window (s).

Time-Restricted feeding is one of the easiest to follow methods of intermittent fasting. Using this along with your daily work and sleep schedule may help achieve optimal metabolic function. Time-restricted feeding is a great program to follow for weight loss and body composition improvements as well as some other overall health benefits. The few human trials that were conducted noted significant reductions in weight, reductions in fasting blood glucose, and improvements in cholesterol with no changes in perceived tension, depression, anger, fatigue, or confusion. Some other preliminary results from animal studies showed time-restricted feeding to protect against obesity, high insulin levels, fatty liver disease, and inflammation.

The easy application and promising results of time-restricted feeding could possibly make it an excellent option for weight loss and chronic disease prevention/management. When implementing this protocol it may be good, to begin with, a lower fasting-to-eating ratio like 12/12 hours and eventually work your way up to 16/8 hours.

Foods For Intermittent Fasting

In this segment, I will like to talk about some foods and will give the advantages they add to the body in their classes. I will start with Harissa

N.B: Before changing the way you eat and altering your diet in any significant way, please speak with a health professional to make sure it's the best decision for you.

HARISSA

Why is this good for you: This spicy chilli paste or powder is having a moment, and for good reason. Recipes for harissa can differ, but in general, they usually contain a mixture of healthy ingredients like chilli peppers, garlic, olive oil and spices. Chilli peppers contain a compound called capsaicin, which is thought to have pain-relief and cancer-protective effects.

How To Eat It: It's super versatile and can be dotted onto fried eggs, mixed into soups or stews, mashed into potatoes— the list goes on. Here's one recipe: Whole Roasted Carrots with Black Lentils and Green Harissa

Nutrition Per 2 Tsp: Calories: 15, Fat: 1 g, Cholesterol: 0 mg,

Sodium: 36 mg, Carbohydrates: 2 g, Dietary fiber: 1 g,

Sugars: 0 g, Protein: 1 g.

GOAT CHEESE

The main reason why it is good for you: Goat cheese can feel indulgent but it actually has less fat per serving than most other cheeses. It also contains protein, calcium and 3% of your daily dose of iron in just an ounce. (Some research has suggested that compared to cow milk, goat milk increases iron absorption and benefits your bones.) Still not convinced? Don't forget that eating for pleasure is good for your health as well.

How To Eat It: However you like it! This recipe combines other healthy superstar

Ingredients too: Quinoa-Stuffed Kale

Rolls with Goat Cheese

Nutrition per 1 ounce: Calories: 103, Fat: 8.5 g, Cholesterol:

22 mg, Sodium: 118 mg, Carbohydrates: 0.03 g, Dietary fiber:

1 g, Sugars: 0.03 g, Protein: 6 g.

POPCORN

Why it's good for you: Popcorn is a high-fibre food that should top your list of go-to snacks. We're not talking about movie theater popcorn, of course. Air-popped popcorn without lots of melted butter and salty seasonings is best.

One study even suggested popcorn is more satisfying than potato chips possibly due to its irregular shape and high volume.

How To Eat It: Try making your popcorn on the stove, it's simple and fast! Instead of butter, sprinkle some parmesan and a little salt.

Nutrition per 1 cup, air-popped: Calories: 31, Fat: 0.4 g,

Cholesterol: 0 mg, Sodium: 1 mg, Carbohydrates: 6 g, Dietary fiber: 1 g, Sugars: 0.07

COCONUT

Why it will be good for you: Coconut is a healthy choice for people with a taste for richness. It has health benefits too. It contains potassium, which can help curb stroke risk, and some research has also shown that adding a little coconut water to rice and letting it cool makes it less caloric.

Coconut water, however, is not a replacement for the real fruit, with some research suggesting the water doesn't always meets its nutritional claims.

How To Eat It: Keep unsweetened shredded coconut in your fridge and sprinkle it on a raw kale or collard green salad.

With tangy vinaigrette on top, it's just delicious, and the small amount of fat it adds makes the salad's nutrients more bioavailable.

Nutrition per 1 cup, shredded: Calories: 283, Fat: 27 g,

Cholesterol: 0 mg, Sodium: 16 mg, Carbohydrates: 12 g,

Dietary fiber: 7 g, Sugars: 5 g, Protein: 2.7 g

GRASS-FED BEEF

Why it is good for you: Grass-fed beef is lower in saturated fat than conventional beef and higher in —good fats‖ such as omega-3s, monounsaturated fatty acids, and conjugated linoleic acid. It's also a great source of protein and iron, which is important for growth and development.

How To Eat It: Whatever cut you like, prepared as you normally would. We also like this:

Grass-Fed Beef Tenderloin

Steaks with Sautéed Mushrooms

Nutrition per 3 ounces: Calories: 99, Fat: 2.3 g, Cholesterol:

47 mg, Sodium: 47 mg, Carbohydrates: 0 g, Dietary fiber: 0 g,

Sugars: 0 g, Protein: 20 g.

GHEE

Why is it helpful to you? Ghee is a clarified butter that is made by melting butter and skimming off some of the fat. It can be easier for some people to digest and is a staple of Indian cuisine. It also has a slightly nutty flavor. It's high in vitamins and can be used as an alternative to cooking oils or butter.

How To Eat It: Use ghee as a cooking tool for a new flavor and a commendable nutritional profile.

Nutrition per 1 tsp: Calories: 45, Fat: 5 g, Cholesterol: 15 mg, Sodium: 0 mg, Carbohydrates:

0 g, Dietary fiber: 0 g,

Sugars: 0 g, Protein: 0 g.

CANNED SALMON

Why it is good for you: Less expensive than fresh salmon, the canned version is one of the richest food sources of vitamin D which is good for bone health and calcium absorption. Its omega-3 fatty acids are another added bonus.

How To Eat It: Canned salmon contains small salmon bones, and you'll definitely want to eat them, they're a great source of calcium that our bodies can more easily absorb than plant sources of calcium. Frying salmon burgers with bread crumbs, eggs, spices, lemon zest and canned salmon, couldn't be easier.

Nutrition per 1 can: Calories: 530, Fat: 20 g, Cholesterol: 226 mg, Sodium: 1656 mg,

Carbohydrates: 0 g, Dietary fiber: 0 g,

Sugars: 0 g, Protein: 60 g.

SPIRULINA

Why it is good for you: Spirulina is a blue-green alga that is high in lots of vitamins, nutrients and antioxidants that protect cells. It's also a good vegetarian source of protein. It can come in pill, powder or flake form, and it is worth doing your research for a trusted variety.

How To Eat It: Add a teaspoon to your morning smoothie or oatmeal.

Nutrition per 1 tbsp: Calories: 20, Fat: 0.5 g, Cholesterol: 0 mg, Sodium: 73 mg,

Carbohydrates: 1.7 g, Dietary fiber: 0.3 g, Sugars: 0.2 g, Protein: 4 g.

LEMON

Why they are good for you: This citrus fruit may be too acidic to eat as you would a milder orange, but it's similarly high in vitamin C, which helps protect cells from damage and is needed by the body to make collagen, which is important for wound healing. Not to mention adding a little lemon zest to any meal adds a flavor kick.

How To Eat It: The easiest way to get vitamin C into your diet without taking pills is to drink lemon water. It's tasty, satisfying and some people swear that if you drink it in the morning, it kickstarts digestion for the day. More evidence is needed, but it can't hurt—and it tastes great.

Nutrition per 1 fruit: Calories: 17, Fat: 0.2 g, Cholesterol: 0 mg, Sodium: 1 mg,

Carbohydrates: 5.4 g, Dietary fiber: 2 g, Sugars: 1.5 g, Protein: 0.6 g.

TOFU

Why it is good for you: Tofu is a great plant-based protein source, and it's high in calcium, protein and iron. Tofu also contains isoflavones, which have benefits related to heart health and a decreased risk of breast and prostate cancer.

How To Eat It: Try the soft kind of tofu that has the consistency of jelly. Its great raw in salads instead of hard-boiled eggs, and you can slice it and dredge in a little egg wash and pan fry for a great appetizer. Top with soy sauce mixed with sesame oil, green onion and black pepper and if you like it spicy, a little sriracha.

Nutrition per 1/2 cup:
Calories: 98,
Fat: 5.3 g,
Cholesterol: 0 mg,
Sodium: 15 mg,
Carbohydrates: 3.6 g,
Dietary fiber: 1 g,
Sugars: 1 g,
Protein: 11.4 g.

DANDELION GREENS

Why they are good for you: Bitter greens like dandelion are rich in vitamin C as well as B vitamins, calcium, iron and potassium. That's an ideal mix for healthy bones and muscles.

How To Eat It: In salads, stewed in stock or like this:

Dandelion-Stuffed Pork Loin

Nutrition per 1 cup, chopped: Calories: 25, Fat: 0.4 g, Cholesterol: 0 mg, Sodium: 42 mg, Carbohydrates: 5 g, Dietary fiber: 2 g, Sugars: 0.4 g, Protein: 1.5 g.

PURPLE POTATOES

Why they are good for you: Like all spud varieties, purple potatoes are rich in potassium — which is needed for blood pressure management. What's special about purple potatoes are their color, which comes from anthocyanin, a potent antioxidant that poses numerous health benefits like a lower risk for cardiovascular disease.

How To Eat It: However you'd eat a regular potato. Or like this: Chilean Beef and Purple Potato Salad.

Nutrition per medium-sized potato: Calories: 93, Fat: 0 g,

Cholesterol: 0 mg, Sodium: 7 mg, Carbohydrates: 20 g,

Dietary fiber: 1 g, Sugars: 0 g, Protein: 3 g.

NUTRITIONAL YEAST

Why it is good for you: Come for the crazy good flavor (nutty, savory and somehow cheesy) and stay for the nutritional punch. Nutritional yeast is a complete protein with all nine essential amino acids as well as zinc, selenium, B vitamins, protein and fiber.

(Nutritional yeast is an inactive yeast that's grown in a culture to make a seasoning rich in nutrients.)

How To Eat It: Some people call this flaky nutritional powerhouse —vegan parmesan‖ but think of it more as a healthy B-vitamin-and-protein-laced umami bomb. It's incredible on popcorn with a little olive oil and some spices.

It's also great as a thickener in pesto, or in any vegetable puree, including cauliflower, mashed potatoes, or —creamed‖ kale or spinach.

Nutrition per ¼ cup: Calories: 60, Fat: 0.5 g,
Cholesterol: 0 mg,
Sodium: 25 mg,
Carbohydrates: 5 g, Dietary fiber: 3 g,

Sugars: 0 g, Protein: 8 g.

OYSTERS

Why They Are Good For You:

Oysters are a great source of protein, omega-3 fatty acids, iron, calcium, zinc, and B12.

Vitamin B12 is important since it keeps the body's nerve and blood cells in good health.

Sadly, the data on their effectiveness as an aphrodisiac is less robust.

How to eat it: Learning how to shuck oysters makes for a great party trick instead of simply offering guests the usual appetizer plate.

Nutrition per 6 mediums: Calories: 43, Fat: 1.4 g,

Cholesterol: 34 mg, Sodium: 71 mg, Carbohydrates: 2.3 g,

Dietary fiber: 0 g, Sugars: 0.5 g, Protein: 5 g.

MANGO

Why it is good for you: This is a very versatile stone fruit, with colors that range from green with a reddish blush to bright yellow. Mangos are also chock full of vitamins and antioxidants, especially vision protective vitamin A: One whole mango provides 45% of your daily value.

How To Eat It: Eat it whole, in a smoothie or in any of Cooking Light's 38 best mango recipes.

Nutrition per 1 fruit: Calories: 202, Fat: 1.3 g,
Cholesterol: 0 mg, Sodium: 3 mg,

Carbohydrates: 50.3 g, Dietary fiber: 5.4g,

Sugars: 46 g, Protein: 2.8 g.

STRAWBERRIES

Why they're good for you: Strawberries are a good source of vitamin C and other compounds involved in metabolism and bone health. They're also high in a subtype of flavonoids called anthocyanins, which are thought to be heart-healthy. A 2013 study of 93,600 women found those who ate more than three or more

servings of 1/2 cup of strawberries or blueberries each week had a lower risk for heart attack.

How to eat it: You don't need our help with this one but here are 20 irresistible strawberry recipes anyway.

Nutrition per 1 cup: Calories: 46, Fat: 0.43 g, Cholesterol: 0 mg, Sodium: 1 mg,

Carbohydrates: 11 g, Dietary fiber: 3 g,

Sugars: 8.1 g, Protein: 1 g.

BLACKBERRIES

Why they are good for you: Blackberries, in particular, are high in fiber, which can increase how full and satisfied you feel after eating, as well as vitamins C, K and manganese.

Research has also linked berry consumption to a wealth of benefits for the body and mind, like lower rates of cognitive decline. The compounds

that make their colors so vibrant can also lower inflammation and support the immune system.

How To Eat It: Bring two cups of steel-cut oats, a pinch of salt, and eight cups of water to a boil. Then turn off the heat, leave it overnight, and top it with blackberries.

Nutrition per 1 cup: Calories: 62, Fat: 0.7 g, Cholesterol: 0 mg, Sodium: 1 mg,

Carbohydrates: 14 g, Dietary fiber: 8 g,

Sugars: 7 g, Protein: 2 g.

ARTICHOKES

Why they are good for you: Artichokes have a meaty texture, and the vegetables are a nutritional powerhouse, rich in folate, dietary fiber, vitamin C, vitamin K and abundant in antioxidants such as quercetin and anthocyanins. When selecting a fresh artichoke to take home, pick one that's heavy and firm (weight is less important with baby artichokes, of course).

How To Eat It: Roasted artichokes take some preparation—you have to remove the tough outer leaves, peel the stem, chop off the top and then soak them in lemon water so they don't brown but the task can be meditative and the result is delicious. Serve with a simple dipping sauce of greek yogurt (or mayo, if you want a treat) mixed with garlic and curry.

Nutrition per 1 medium artichoke: Calories: 60, Fat: 0.2 g,

Cholesterol: 0 mg, Sodium: 120 mg, Carbohydrates: 13.5 g,

Dietary fiber: 7 g, Sugars: 1.3 g, Protein: 4.2 g.

SAUERKRAUT

Why it is good for you: Sauerkraut is fermented cabbage that contains fiber and multiple vitamins that make it a good addition to your dinner plate. Sauerkraut is a good source of iron, manganese, copper, sodium, magnesium, and calcium. Not to mention it contributes a moderate amount of protein to your diet. Like other fermented foods, sauerkraut contains probiotics that benefit the gut and digestion.

How To Eat It: You can do the fermenting yourself with this recipe for Red Sauerkraut or buy it pre-made and eat it on its own, with eggs, or mixed into salads or slaws.

Nutrition per 1 cup: Calories: 27, Fat: 0.2 g, Cholesterol: 0 mg, Sodium: 939 mg,

Carbohydrates: 6.1 g, Dietary fiber: 4 g,

Sugars: 3 g, Protein: 1.3 g.

SPAGHETTI SQUASH

Why it is good for you: Spaghetti squash has one of the highest water contents of all the winter squash. It's low in calories and can be used to substitute pasta in many recipes. It also yields a good dose of vitamin A, calcium, vitamin C and fiber.

How To Eat It: Substitute it for pasta in your favorite dish. It won't look exactly the same, but you'll get a delicious vegetable overload. You can also strain them and form them into patties that you bake in the oven.

Nutrition per 1 cup: Calories: 42, Fat: 0.4 g, Cholesterol: 0mg, Sodium: 28 mg,

Carbohydrates: 10 g, Dietary fiber: 2 g, Sugars: 4 g, Protein: 1 g.

APPLES

Why they are good for you: There's a reason —an apple a day‖ is a thing. Apples are rich in a type of fiber that can lower cholesterol levels, making them a heart-healthy snack. One study found eating apples led people to eat 15% fewer calories at their next meal. Another perk? They're helpful for regulating digestion.

How To Eat It: Fry up some kale and then saute it with garlic and diced apples.

Nutrition per 1 medium apple: Calories: 95, Fat: 0.3 g,

Cholesterol: 0 mg, Sodium: 2 mg, Carbohydrates: 25 g,

Dietary fiber: 4 g, Sugars: 19 g, Protein: 0.5 g.

WILD CAUGHT COD

Why it's good for you: Wild caught cod is a versatile and sustainable fish that is available throughout the year. Though the fish is lower in fat, a high percentage of its fat comes in the form of omega-3 fatty acids, which are associated with a decreased risk of cardiovascular disease.

How To Eat It: Mix up a miso-based marinade and roast it in the oven.

Nutrition per 3 ounces: Calories: 71, Fat: 0.2 g, Cholesterol:

52 mg, Sodium: 114 mg, Carbohydrates: 0 g, Protein: 17.4 g.

RHUBARB

Why it is good for you: Few leafy foods look as lovely as rhubarb with its deep red stalks and bright green leaves (just remember not to eat the latter, as they're poisonous). It's high in vitamins and folate, as well.

How To Eat It: Forget jam or pie try pickling your rhubarb for a savory kick.

Nutrition per 1 stalk: Calories: 11, Fat: 0.1 g, Cholesterol: 0 mg, Sodium: 2 mg,

Carbohydrates: 2.3 g, Dietary fiber: 1 g,

Sugars: 0.6 g, Protein: 0.5 g.

BEET GREENS

Why they are good for you: It's hard to compete with the deep reds of beets, but don't toss the greens that sprout from them. The leaves of some beets, like golden and Chioggia varieties (which are striped on the inside!) are especially lush and thick and can be tossed into salads. They're high in vitamin A and vitamin K, and a cup boasts 44 mg of calcium.

How To Eat It: Beet Soup with Potatoes and Beet Greens

Nutrition per 1 cup: Calories: 8, Fat: 0.05 g, Cholesterol: 0 mg, Sodium: 86 mg,

Carbohydrates: 1.7 g, Dietary fiber: 1.4 g,
Sugars: 0.2 g, Protein: 0.8 g.

PURPLE CAULIFLOWER

Why it is good for you: Like purple potatoes, the unexpected shade of this cauliflower comes from the antioxidant anthocyanin. Cauliflower is low in calories and rich in fiber, vitamin C, folate, manganese, vitamin K and B6 (which is involved in metabolism and early brain development). Consider steaming or stir-frying cauliflower to keep nutrient levels high.

How To Eat It: Steamed or roasted at 400 °F and then pureed. Add a glug of olive oil, salt and pepper, and at the end, toss in any fresh herbs you may have, such as thyme, rosemary or even mint and basil. Consider it a healthier and more elevated mashed potato.

Nutrition per 1 cup, chopped: Calories: 27, Fat: 0.3 g,

Cholesterol: 0 mg, Sodium: 32 mg, Carbohydrates: 5.3 g,

Dietary fiber: 2 g, Sugars: 2 g, Protein: 2.1 g.

ENDIVE

Why it is good for you: Endive is high in inulin and fiber; which can lower LDL cholestrol levels to benefit the heart. Endive is also a great source of vitamin A and beta-carotene as well as B vitamins, iron and potassium. Often used raw in salads or appetizers, cooked endive can taste sweet and nutty.

How To Eat It: Bacon Endive Tomato Bites

Nutrition per 1 cup, chopped: Calories: 8, Fat: 0.1 g,

Cholesterol: 0 mg, Sodium: 11 mg, Carbohydrates: 1.7 g,

Dietary fiber: 1.6 g, Sugars: 0.1 g, Protein: 0.6 g.

SNAP PEAS

Why they are good for you: Small veggies are ideal snacks on the go since they're high in nutrients and fiber and they taste great raw. A good snap pea should look moist—when they are dry they taste starchy. They're also high in vitamins A, K, and C.

How To Eat It: Snap peas are delicious plain or dipped into hummus, but if you want to mix it up a bit, drizzle some red wine vinegar or rice vinegar on top of them, mixed with a little oil, and serve.

Nutrition per 1 cup: Calories: 31, Fat: 0.2 g, Cholesterol: 0 mg, Sodium: 6 mg,

Carbohydrates: 7 g, Dietary fiber: 3 g,

Sugars: 3.3 g, Protein: 2 g.

CORN

Why it is good for you: There may be no other vegetable more evocative of summer than corn, though there are certainly reasons to eat it year-round. One ear of corn has approximately the same calories as an apple, with equally high nutrient levels, too. Non-genetically modified corn is also loaded with lutein and zeaxanthin, two phytochemicals that promote healthy vision.

How To Eat It: Oaxacan-Style Grilled Corn on the Cob

Nutrition per 1 medium ear: Calories: 99, Fat: 1.5 g,

Cholesterol: 0 mg, Sodium: 1 mg, Carbohydrates: 22 g,

Dietary fiber: 3 g, Sugars: 5 g, Protein: 4 g.

PUMPKIN

Why it is good for you: Pumpkin is not just for carving. Its seeds are high in potassium and magnesium, and pumpkin flesh is rich in beta-carotene, which is good for the immune system. One cup of canned pumpkin contains 7g fiber and 3 grams of protein, which is helpful for regular digestion.

Pumpkin also contains 50% of the daily value of vitamin K, which helps prevent blood clotting.

How To Eat It: Make a toasted pumpkin seed pesto. Throw them in a food processor with basil, olive oil, parmesan, garlic and lemon juice. Or roast, puree and eat it as a side dish or mixed in with potatoes.

Nutrition per 1 cup mashed: Calories: 49, Fat: 0.2 g,

Cholesterol: 0 mg, Sodium: 2 mg, Carbohydrates: 12 g,

Dietary fiber: 3 g, Sugars: 5 g, Protein: 1.8 g.

KIMCHI

Why it is good for you: Kimchi is the Korean version of fermented cabbage and is loaded with vitamin A, B vitamins and vitamin C. Similar to sauerkraut, it contains healthy probiotics that regulate digestion. It adds a kick of flavour to almost any recipe.

How To Eat It: You can buy it or make it yourself. It tastes great by the spoonful, or you can try it in a recipe like Kimchi Jjigae (Kimchi-Pork Soup).

Nutrition per 1 cup: Calories: 22, Fat: 0.8 g, Cholesterol: 0 mg, Sodium: 747 mg,

Carbohydrates: 4 g, Dietary fiber: 2.4 g,

Sugars: 1.6 g, Protein: 1.7 g.

OLIVES

Why they are good for you: We know olive oil is a common ingredient in a healthy diet, but don't forget about its source.

Olives are high in healthy fat that can benefit your heart and brain and keep weight in check. Research has also suggested that olives are a good source of antioxidants that prevent the buildup of bad cholesterol in artery walls.

They're also a fermented food, and therefore are good sources of gut-friendly bacteria.

How To Eat It: Pour them into a dish and serve, or slice them up and add them to any pasta recipe.

Nutrition per 1 large olive: Calories: 5, Fat: 0.5 g,

Cholesterol: 0 mg, Sodium: 32 mg, Carbohydrates: 0.3 g,

Dietary fiber: 0.1 g, Sugars: 0 g, Protein: 0 g.

ASPARAGUS

Why it is good for you: Asparagus is a good source of folate, which is essential for a wide variety of body functions, as well as vitamins A, C and K. When purchasing asparagus, avoid spears with smashed tips, which will spoil more easily.

How To Eat It: Use a peeler to cut asparagus into little ribbons to mix into salads. Also, try them oven roasted whole at 375

°F for 12 minutes and then served with sunny side up eggs for breakfast. There's something really fun about poking egg yolks with an asparagus spear.

Nutrition per 1 spear: Calories: 3, Fat: 0 g, Cholesterol: 0 mg, Sodium: 0 mg, Carbohydrates:

0.6 g, Dietary fiber: 0.3 g,

Sugars: 0.3 g, Protein: 0.4 g.

FIGS

Why they are good for you: This fruit is high in both vitamins A and C, and have a unique taste that allows flexibility for both sweet and savoury dishes. Avoid figs with bruises, but they should be a bit soft when you're choosing which ones to bring home.

How To Eat It: Pair them with healthy appetizers like almonds and cheese for your guests, or get cooking with these 20

Fantastic Fig Recipes.

Nutrition per 1 fig: Calories: 37, Fat: 0.2 g, Cholesterol: 0 mg, Sodium: 0 mg, Carbohydrates:

9.6 g, Dietary fiber: 1.4 g,

Sugars: 8 g, Protein: 0.4 g.

KOHLRABI

Why it is good for you: This peculiar-looking root vegetable has a pale green or purple bulb which sprouts multiple stalks with dark leaves–and you can eat all its parts. Kohlrabi is a cousin to broccoli and cauliflower and is high in fibre and potassium.

How to eat it: They taste greatly roasted in olive oil or nestled under a roast chicken as it cooks. You can also try Honey Glazed Kohlrabi with Onions and Herbs.

Nutrition per 1 cup: Calories: 36, Fat: 0.1 g, Cholesterol: 0 mg, Sodium: 27 mg,

Carbohydrates: 8.4 g, Dietary fiber: 5 g, Sugars: 4 g, Protein: 2 g.

PORK TENDERLOIN

Why it is good for you: Pork tenderloin is now certified with the American Heart Association ―heart check‖ mark, indicating it qualifies as an extra-lean and heart-healthy meat. Additionally, it is an excellent source of protein, B vitamins and zinc.

How To Eat It: 18 Light Pork Loin Recipes

Nutrition per 3 ounces: Calories: 159, Fat: 5.4 g,

Cholesterol: 1 mg, Sodium: 55 mg, Carbohydrates: 0 g,

Dietary fiber: 0 g, Protein: 26 g.

COFFEE

Why it is good for you: There has been back and forth on how much is too much when it comes to the morning cup. But one study of 130,000 adults found no evidence that coffee increases the risk for health problems like heart disease or cancer, even among people who drank 48-ounces a day. The fact is, coffee is a complex drink containing hundreds of different compounds. Some of those include antioxidants that have been linked to a lower risk for type 2 diabetes, Alzheimer's and liver cancer, Romano says. Keep in mind, that's without added sugar and cream.

How To Eat It: Brew yourself a cup in the morning and drink it as plain as possible—the health benefits come from the coffee, not the cream and sugar you add to it.

Nutrition per 1 cup: Calories: 5, Fat: 0 g, Cholesterol: 0 mg,

Sodium: 2 mg, Carbohydrates: 0.6 g, Dietary fiber: 0 g,

Sugars: 0 g, Protein: 0.7 g.

KOMBUCHA

Why it is good for you: This fermented drink is rich in probiotics, which benefit the healthy bacteria in your gut, aid in digestion, and increase the absorption of nutrients in food

How to eat it: Kombucha is increasingly becoming an easy-to-find beverage at the grocery.

Nutrition per bottle: Calories: 33, Fat: 0 g, Cholesterol: 0 mg, Sodium: 10 mg, Carbohydrates:

7 g, Sugars: 2 g, Protein: 0 g.

BUCKWHEAT

Why it is good for you: This whole grain, which is also gluten-free, is rich in fiber and is a complete protein. (Fun fact: it's what's used to make soba noodles.)

How To Eat It: It can be used as the base for a dish instead of rice, in soups or in tasty baked goods like Buckwheat Belgian Waffles.

Nutrition per 1 cup: Calories: 583, Fat: 5.8

g, Cholesterol: 0 mg, Sodium: 2 mg,

Carbohydrates: 121.6 g, Dietary fiber: 17 g, Protein: 23 g.

GINGER ROOT

Why it is good for you: This twisted root is a natural remedy for nausea and motion sickness and has been used in traditional medicine for thousands of years. Not only does it pack a zingy flavor, it also contains compounds like beta-carotene and capsaicin, which provide all sorts of healing and immune supportive wonders to the body.

How To Eat It: If you're worried about having to buy a whole root and only using a little bit, wrap it and store in the freezer. Take it out and micro plane it onto fish, chicken, salad dressings, or anywhere you need a little zing.

Nutrition per 5 small slices: Calories: 9, Fat: 0.1 g,

Cholesterol: 0 mg, Sodium: 1 mg, Carbohydrates: 2 g, Dietary fiber: 0.2 g, Sugars: 0.2 g,

Protein: 0.2 g.

TAHINI

Why it is good for you: Tahini, which is made from ground sesame seeds, is a good way get in some calcium, iron, potassium and vitamin E. Just one tablespoon has 110 mg of phosphorus, too, which is critical for the formation of bones and teeth. It also works with B vitamins to help with nerve signalling, normal heartbeat, and muscle contractions.

How To Eat It: Tahini is a great base for salad dressings and marinades for fish. It's also a key ingredient in hummus.

Nutrition per 1 tbsp: Calories: 89, Fat: 8 g, Cholesterol: 0 mg, Sodium: 17 mg,

Carbohydrates: 3.2 g, Dietary fiber: 1.4 g, Sugars: 0.1 g, Protein: 3 g.

BASIL

Why it is good for you: Basil, which is actually a member of the mint family, is the star ingredient in pesto. The oil extracts from basil leaves contain antioxidant compounds that combat inflammation. Also high in vitamins, it's a simple way to add a touch of nutrition to many recipes, and it pairs well with hearty vegetables.

How To Eat It: You cannot go wrong tossing it into Asian stir-fries, onto pasta or pizza, and shredding it into salad. Tear or cut just before serving, and check out Cooking Light's Guide to Basil.

Nutrition per 5 leaves: Calories: 1, Fat: 0.02 g, Cholesterol: 0 mg, Sodium: 0 mg,

Carbohydrates: 0.07 g, Dietary fiber: 0 g,

Sugars: 0 g, Protein: 0.08 g.

PISTACHIOS

Why they are good for you: In addition to their heart-healthy fats, pistachios are rich in antioxidants, including lutein, beta-carotene and gamma-tocopherol. They are also high in vitamin A, which is important for vision and proper organ function.

They're delicious and surprisingly light for a nut: 50kernels are only around 160 calories.

How To Eat It: Keep pistachios in the fridge so you can regularly chop them up and toss them into salads, on top of roasted broccoli, and even into soups.

Nutrition per 1 ounce serving: Calories: 159, Fat: 13 g,

Cholesterol: 0 mg, Sodium: 0 mg, Carbohydrates: 8 g,
Dietary fiber: 3 g, Sugars: 2.2 g,
Protein: 6 g.

SPELT

Why it is good for you: Spelt is becoming an increasingly popular grain due to its nutritional profile. Spelt includes complex carbohydrates and is rich in both soluble and insoluble fiber, vitamin B2, niacin, manganese, thiamin, copper and magnesium. It even has fatty and amino acids, which are important for body function.

How To Eat It: Try this: Spelt and Wild Mushroom Soup with Pasta.

Nutrition per serving: (one cup cooked) Calories: 246, Fat: 2 g, Cholesterol: 0 mg, Sodium:

1. mg, Carbohydrates: 51.3 g, Dietary fiber: 8 g, Protein: 11 g.

SUNFLOWER SEEDS

Why they are good for you: Seeds, like sunflower seeds, for example, are high in vitamin E which has antioxidant activity that's good for immunity functions.

One ounce of dry-roasted sunflower seeds contains 7.4 mg of vitamin E, which is 37% of your daily value.

How To Eat Them: Toss them on top of salads, in oatmeal, or pour a handful into a baggie and eat them as a snack.

Nutrition per 1 ounce: Calories: 165, Fat: 14 g, Cholesterol:

0 mg, Sodium: 1 mg, Carbohydrates: 7 g, Dietary fiber: 3 g,

Sugars: 1 g, Protein: 5.5 g.

WATER

Even though you are not eating, it is important to stay hydrated for so many reasons, like the health of basically every major organ in your body. The amount of water that any one person should drink varies, but you want your urine to be a pale yellow color at all times. Dark yellow urine indicates dehydration, which can cause headaches, fatigue, and lightheadedness.

Couple that with limited food, and it could be a recipe for disaster. If the thought of plain water doesn't excite you, add a squeeze of lemon juice, a few mint leaves, or cucumber slices to your water. It'll be our little secret.

On this, I love to include sports drinks because this is also needed to boost your energy levels. Hydration is a major factor as a significant amount of water is lost through sweat during a workout. But drinking water immediately afterwards is not recommended, as it will cool your body instantly. Because one must slowly rebuild the water loss after a workout. It advisable to consume half a litre of water in 2 hours before workout, and for this rebuilding one needs to take 250ml of water during the warm-up time or period, and 150-200ml every 20-30 minutes during the session.

Healthy Exercise To Support Intermittent Fasting

I will also like to give some tips on some exercises that can mostly benefit women.

One in four women experiences pelvic floor problems which can lead to incontinence or even prolapse. Pelvic floor exercises are designed to strengthen the pelvic floor, the sling of muscles that support the bladder, bowel and uterus which can weaken with ageing and after childbirth.

Exercises can be done sitting down, standing up, or lying down, and involve actively tightening and lifting your pelvic floor muscles at different intervals.

i. A Pelvic floor physiotherapist professional once said women should start in a comfortable position and follow the steps below:

ii. Squeeze the muscles around the front of your pelvis, imagine you are stopping urination then squeezing the vaginal walls together

iii. Pull up through the back passage as if you are stopping wind

iv. Let go

v. Do this ten times at maximum capacity without allowing other muscles to help

Once this is mastered, a professional said: —women should move on to pelvic floor endurance exercise.
"You do the same exercise but hold it a little less intensely and hold it over a longer period of time," the professional says. "It is like going for a jog instead of a sprint."

i. Hold the position (as detailed above) for ten seconds in a relaxed state

ii. Finish with ten quick pulses to get quick fiber moving

iii. Repeat ten times, professional in this aspect said quick pulses help to turn the pelvic floor on for things like sneezing, coughing and jumping.

"If you get this done most days and commit to it at least twice a day, you will notice amazing results." she said. She added by saying because many women have difficulty locating the right muscles and practising the correct technique, it may be helpful to work with a pelvic floor physiotherapist or nurse. Over time, strengthening these muscles with regular exercise can help women prevent pelvic floor weakness and reduce symptoms of prolapse.

Another way to help an individual are these and all these will be elucidated more after the ten exercises are explained.

JUMP ROPE

This is a perfect cardio move, plus it is a great calf exercise. It warms up the body, it also strengthens the muscles, it increases aerobic fitness and burns a lot of calories in a little period. Though some looks or see it as a play, this is beyond that.

QUICK FEET

For this, if your goal is to improve your speed and agility, and get a good cardio boost while working your lower body, try adding the quick feet exercise to your workout routine.

MOUNTAIN CLIMBERS

Mountain climbers are a dynamic, compound exercise and an all-over leg strengthener. The jumping movement strengthens your calves, abs, thighs, glutes and hips.

WALL SIT PLIES CALF RAISE

This exercise aims at strengthening your inner and outer thighs, calves, quads, hamstrings, glutes and hips, it also engages your core and lower back, to help keep your body balanced and steady which is the aim of everyone that engages in this exercise.

INVERTED V PLANK

The inverted v plank is a bodyweight exercise that strengthens and tones your core, glutes, shoulders, thighs and calves. Inverted v plank puts your whole body to work, improves your stability and flexibility, and boosts the metabolism.

BASKETBALL SHOT

The basketball shot is a high impact, full body exercise that improves aerobic fitness, builds strength, and increases speed and coordination. This move targets the legs, core, glutes and shoulders, boosts the metabolism and improves stamina and endurance.

TOUCH AND HOP

The touch and hop is a full body cardio move that challenges your balance and stability and improves strength, power and agility. This exercise strengthens your legs, boosts the metabolism and maximizes weight loss.

ANKLE HOPS

Ankle hops tone and sculpt the legs, strengthen the heart and muscles, and increase aerobic fitness. This exercise also boosts your agility, coordination and speed.

CALF RAISES

Calf raises target, as the name implies, your calves. This exercise increases muscle strength, allowing you to jump higher, and improves the tone, definition, and appearance of the lower legs.

PLIE SQUAT CALF RAISE

The plie squat with calf raise is a great exercise to strengthen your legs and glutes. This exercise targets the muscles in the back of the lower legs, your calves, but due to the plie squat position.

All these ten exercises will help if you want your legs to look amazing in high heels, you need to start paying special attention to your calves. Strong and sculpted legs not only look fabulous in a short dress but can also help you boost your athletic performance and provide your body with a solid foundation to build on. And the addition of these ten exercise on your leg workout, engage your calves and feet the burn.

CHAPTER THREE

HEALTHY RECIPES FOR INTERMITTENT FASTING

About The Recipes

These recipes are easy to make and designed for 5:2 (2 fast days and 5 days where you eat normally) restricted days as part of an intermittent diet and should form your diet for no more than two (ideally consecutive) days of any week. These recipes are low-calorie recipes that you can enjoy on your fasting days that will leave you feeling full and satisfied. All the recipes are easy to adapt to your own taste.

Adapting The Recipes To Suit You

All of the recipes in this article are very adaptable. If you change any of the ingredients though it's important to still know how many calories you are eating, so you will need to do your own research to find out the amount of calories per amount of food you are eating.

LIGHTER CREAMY MUSHROOMS ON TOAST

Preparation Time Cooking Time Serves

Less Than 30 Minutes

Less Than 10 Minutes

Serves 1

So creamy and luxurious you will never realize this breakfast is only 200 kcal and counts as one of your five a day.

NUTRITIONAL VALUE PER SERVING

Each serving provides 200 kcal, 17g protein, 14g carbohydrate (of which 3g sugars), 8g fat (of which 3g saturates), 3g fiber and 1.4g salt

INGREDIENTS

- 1 tsp rapeseed oil
- 80g/3oz button mushrooms, roughly chopped
- 32g/1oz reduced-fat smoked bacon medallion, roughly chopped,
- 2 spring onions, thinly sliced
- 1 garlic clove, finely chopped
- ½ small lemon, juice only
- 1 level tbsp half-fat crème fraîche
- 30g/1oz slice wholemeal or granary bread
- salt and freshly ground black pepper, to taste

- 1 tbsp chopped fresh chives (optional)

METHOD

1. Heat the oil in small frying pan over a medium heat. Add the mushrooms, bacon, and spring onions and garlic and cook for 1–2 minutes. Add the lemon juice, then cover with a lid and cook over a low heat for 5 minutes, or until the mushrooms are cooked.

2. Remove from the heat, stir in the crème fraîche and chives, if using, and season.

3. Toast the bread on both sides, place on a warmed plate and top with the mushrooms.

BANANA MUFFINS

Preparation time less than 30 minutes

Cooking time 10 to 30 minutes

Serves

Makes 6 muffins

Ripe bananas add sweetness to muffins, so you don't have to use much sugar. Wholemeal flour gives the muffins plenty of fiber, keeping you full for longer.

NUTRITIONAL VALUE PER SERVING

Each muffin provides 206 kcal, 4.5g protein, 30g carbohydrate (of which 13g sugars), 7.5g fat (of which 0.8g saturates), 1g fiber and 0.4 salt

INGREDIENTS

- 125g/4½oz wholemeal flour
- 3 level tbsp light muscovite sugar
- 2 level tsp baking powder
- 1 medium free-range egg, beaten
- 50g/1¾oz low-fat plain yoghurt
- 50ml/2fl oz rapeseed oil, plus a little extra for greasing
- 2 ripe bananas (175g/6oz peeled weight), roughly mashed

METHOD

1. Preheat the oven to 200C/180C Fan/Gas 6. Line a six-hole muffin tin with muffin cases or grease it.

2. Mix together the flour, sugar and baking powder in a bowl. In a separate bowl, beat together the egg, yoghurt and oil. Make a well in the flour, pour in the liquid and mix well. Stir in the mashed bananas, taking care not to over-mix.

3. Spoon the mixture into the prepared cases and bake for 20–30 minutes, or until a skewer inserted into the centre comes out clean. Transfer the muffins to a wire rack to cool.

Recipe Tips: These muffins freeze well, so make a batch and freeze for up to three months.

GARLIC MUSHROOM FRITTATA

Preparation time less than 30 minutes

Cooking time 10 to 30 minutes

Serves 2

Garlic and mushrooms bring great flavor to this super low calorie, easy to make frittata.

Serve with salad for a simple and delicious lunch.

NUTRITIONAL VALUE PER SERVING

As part of an intermittent diet plan, 1 serving provides 3 of your 6 daily vegetable portions. This meal provides 243 kcal, 14grams protein, 3.5grams carbohydrate (of which 3grams sugars), 14grams fat (of which 4grams saturates), 2.5grams fiber and 0.6gram salt per portion.

INGREDIENTS

- Low-calorie cooking spray
- 250g/9oz chestnut mushrooms, sliced
- 1 small garlic clove, crushed
- 1 tbsp thinly sliced fresh chives
- 4 large free-range eggs, beaten
- freshly ground black pepper

FOR THE SALAD

- 1 Little Gem lettuce leaves separated
- 100g/3½oz cherry tomatoes halved
- 1/3 cucumber, cut into chunks

METHOD

1. Spray a small, flame-proof frying pan with oil and place over a high heat. (The base of the pan shouldn't be wider than about 18cm/7in.) Stir-fry the mushrooms in three batches for 2-3 minutes, or until softened and lightly browned. Tip the cooked mushrooms into a sieve over a bowl to catch any juices – you don't want the mushrooms to become soggy.

2. Return all the mushrooms to the pan and stir in the garlic and chives, and a pinch of ground black pepper. Cook for a further minute, then reduces the heat to low.

3. Preheat the grill to its hottest setting. Pour the eggs over the mushrooms. Cook for five minutes, or until almost set.

4. Place the pan under the grill for 3-4 minutes, or until set.

5. Combine the salad ingredients in a bowl.

6. Remove from the grill and loosen the sides of the frittata with a round-bladed knife. Turn out onto a board and cut into wedges. Serve hot or cold with the salad.

CHICKEN AND VEGETABLE BALTI

Preparation time less than 30 minutes

Cooking time 30 minutes to 1 hour

Serves Serves 2

Try this chicken and vegetable balti for a healthy curry that is quick and easy to prepare.

NUTRITIONAL VALUE PER SERVING

As part of an intermittent diet plan, 1 serving provides 1 of your 3 daily low-fat dairy portions 2 of your 6 daily vegetable portions. This meal provides 341 kcal, 40g protein, 30.5g carbohydrate (of which 20.5g sugars), 6g fat (of which 1.5grams saturates), 9g fiber and 0.6g salt per portion.

INGREDIENTS

- Calorie controlled cooking oil spray
- 1 medium onion, thinly sliced
- 4 chicken thighs, boned and skinned
- 1 red pepper, deseeded and cut into 3cm/1in chunks
- 1 yellow pepper, deseeded and cut into 3cm/1in chunks
- 1 tbsp corn flour
- 150g/5½oz fat-free natural yogurt
- 1 tbsp medium or mild curry powder
- 2 garlic cloves, thinly sliced
- 227g/8oz tin chopped tomatoes
- 3 heaped tbsp finely chopped fresh coriander, plus extra to garnish
- freshly ground black pepper

METHOD

1. Spray a large, deep, non-stick frying pan or wok with oil and place over a medium heat. Add the onion and cook for five minutes, stirring regularly until well softened and lightly browned.

2. Meanwhile, trim all the visible fat off the chicken thighs, cut each one into four pieces and season with black pepper.

3. Add the chicken and peppers into the pan with the onion and cook for three minutes, turning occasionally.

4. Meanwhile, in a small bowl, mix the cornflour with 2 tablespoons cold water and stir in the yoghurt until thoroughly mixed.

5. Sprinkle the curry powder over the chicken and vegetables, add the garlic and cook for 30 seconds.

6. Tip the tomatoes into the pan, add the yoghurt mixture, 150ml/3½fl oz of water and coriander.

7. Bring to a gentle simmer and cook for 20-25 minutes, stirring occasionally until the chicken is tender and the sauce is thick. Season with freshly ground black pepper to taste and garnish with coriander.

CRUNCHY BANANA YOGHURT

Preparation time : - less than 30 minutes

Cooking time: - no cooking required

Serves: - Serves 2

Banana and yoghurt are a perfect low-calorie breakfast combination that will keep you going until lunchtime. The banana adds sweetness without the need for extra sugar and the seeds bring a satisfying crunch. As part of an intermittent diet plan.

NUTRITIONAL VALUE PER SERVING

1 serving provides your daily piece of fruit 2 of your 3 daily low-fat dairy portions. This meal provides 149 kcal per portion.

INGREDIENTS

- 340g/12oz fat-free natural Greek-style yoghurt

- 1 banana, peeled and sliced

- 15g/½oz mixed seeds (pumpkin, sesame and sunflower) (or use toasted flaked almonds)

METHOD

1. Divide the yoghurt between two small bowls. Scatter the banana on top.

2. Sprinkle with seeds or nuts and serve.

RECIPE TIPS

Look out for mixed bags of pumpkin, sesame and sunflower seeds but watch your portion size carefully as they are very high in calories.

CAPONATA RATATOUILLE

Preparation time less than 30 minutes

Cooking time 30 minutes to 1 hour

Serves Serves 6

Ratatouille is a wonderfully warming vegetable stew originating from Provence. Perfect for pleasing vegetables and meat eaters alike.

NUTRITIONAL VALUE PER SERVING

Your daily salty food 2 of your 6 daily vegetable portions. This meal provides 90 kcal per portion.

INGREDIENTS

- 1 tbsp olive oil
- 750g/1lb 10oz aborigines, cut into 1cm/1½in chunks
- 1 large onion, cut into 1cm/1½in chunks3 celery sticks, roughly chopped
- 2 large beef tomatoes, skinned and deseeded
- 1 tsp chopped thyme
- ¼-½ tsp cayenne pepper
- 2 tbsp capers, drained
- small handful of pitted green olives
- 4 tbsp white wine vinegar
- 1 tbsp sugar
- 1-2 tbsp cocoa powder (optional)

- freshly ground black pepper
- To garnish
- chopped almonds, toasted
- chopped parsley

METHOD

1. Heat the oil in a non-stick frying pan until very hot, add the aborigine and fry for about 15 minutes, or until very soft. Add a little boiling water to prevent sticking if necessary.

2. Meanwhile, place the onion and celery in a large saucepan with a little water. Cook for 5 minutes, or until tender but still firm.

3. Add the tomatoes, thyme, cayenne pepper and aborigine to the saucepan. Cook for 15 minutes, stirring occasionally. Add the capers, olives, vinegar, sugar and cocoa powder and cook for 2-3 minutes.

4. Season with freshly ground black pepper. Divide between 6 bowls, garnish with the toasted almonds and parsley and serve.

ITALIAN STYLE MEATBALLS WITH COURGETTE 'TAGLIATELLE'

Preparation time less than 30 minutes

Cooking time 10 to 30 minutes

Serves Serves 2

This flavorful dish of Italian meatballs has a healthy twist by using coquette ribbons instead of pasta, an easy way to reduce calories.

NUTRITIONAL VALUE PER SERVING

As part of an intermittent diet plan, 1 serving provides 3 of your 6 daily vegetable portions.
This meal provides 219 kcal per portion.

INGREDIENTS

FOR THE MEATBALLS
- 250g/9oz extra lean beef mince (5% fat or less)
- 1 small onion, very finely chopped
- 1 tsp dried mixed herbs
- calorie controlled cooking oil spray
- 1 garlic clove, crushed
- 227g/8oz can chopped tomatoes
- 2 heaped tbsp finely shredded fresh basil leaves, plus extra to garnish

FOR THE COURGETTE _TAGLIATELLE'
- 2 medium courgettes, trimmed and deseeded

- sea salt and freshly ground black pepper

METHOD

1. Place the beef, half the onion, half the mixed herbs and a pinch of salt and pepper in a bowl and mix well. Form into 10 small balls.

2. Spray a medium non-stick frying pan with a little oil and cook the meatballs for 5-7 minutes, turning occasionally until browned on all sides. Transfer to a plate.

3. For the sauce, put the remaining onion in the same pan and cook over a low heat for three minutes, stirring. Add the garlic and cook for a few seconds.

4. Stir in the tomatoes, 300ml/10fl oz water, the remaining mixed herbs and shredded basil. Bring to the boil, stirring. Return the meatballs to the pan, reduce the heat to a simmer and cook for 20 minutes, stirring occasionally until the sauce is thick and the meatballs are cooked throughout.

5. Meanwhile, half-fill a medium pan with water and bring to the boil. Use a vegetable peeler to peel the courgettes into ribbons. Cook the courgette in the boiling water for one minute then drain.

6. Divide the courgette ribbons between two plates and top with the meatballs and sauce. Garnish with basil leaves.

CHERMOULA TOFU AND ROASTED VEGETABLES

Preparation time less than 30 minutes

Cooking time 30 minutes to 1 hour

Serves Serves 4

Tofu wonderfully absorbs the flavours of chermoula in this dish. Serve with roasted vegetables for a hearty vegetarian meal.

NUTRITIONAL VALUE PER SERVING

As part of an intermittent diet plan, 1 serving provides 2 of your daily vegetable portions.
This meal provides 182 kcal per portion.

INGREDIENTS

FOR THE CHERMOULA TOFU
- 25g/1oz coriander, finely chopped
- 3 garlic cloves, chopped
- 1 tsp cumin seeds, lightly crushed
- 1 lemon, finely grated rind
- ½ tsp dried crushed chillies
- 1 tbsp olive oil
- 250g/9oz tofu

FOR THE ROASTED VEGETABLES
- 2 red onions, quartered
- 2 courgettes, thickly sliced

- 2 red peppers, deseeded and sliced
- 2 yellow peppers, deseeded and sliced
- 1 small aubergine, thickly sliced
- low-calorie cooking spray
- pinch salt

METHOD

1. Preheat the oven to 200C/180C Fan/ Gas 6.

2. For the chermoula, mix the coriander, garlic, cumin, lemon rind and chilies together with the oil and a little salt in a small bowl.

3. Pat the tofu dry on kitchen paper and cut it in half. Cut each half horizontally into thin slices. Spread the chermoula generously over the slices.

4. Scatter the vegetables in a roasting tin and spray with oil. Bake for about 45 minutes, until lightly browned, turning the ingredients once or twice during cooking.

5. Arrange the tofu slices over the vegetables, with the side spread with the chermoula uppermost, and bake for a further 10-15 minutes, or until the tofu is lightly colored.

6. Divide the tofu and vegetables between four plates and serve.

BERRY YOGHURT

Preparation time less than 30 minutes

Cooking time no cooking required

Serves Serves 2

A Luscious, fruity yogurt that makes a satisfying breakfast, Using frozen berries saves money and they make a delicious juice as they thaw.

NUTRITIONAL VALUE PER SERVING

As part of an intermittent diet plan, 1 serving provides your daily piece of fruit 2 of your 3 daily low-fat dairy portions. This meal provides 149 kcal per portion.

INGREDIENTS

- 175g/6oz frozen mixed berries, defrosted
- 340g/12oz fat-free Greek yoghurt
- 10g/¼oz flaked almonds, toasted

METHOD

1. Spoon the yoghurt into two glasses, top with half the berries, and then repeat the layers.
2. Sprinkle with the flaked almonds and serve.

Recipe Tips

You can toast the almonds in a dry frying pan or buy the ready toasted kind.

HEARTY VEGETABLE SOUP

Preparation time less than 30 minutes

Cooking time 30 minutes to 1 hour

Serves Serves 2

This hearty vegetable soup is packed full of flavor and goodness, perfect to warm you up on a cold night. If eating on a restricted day of an intermittent diet, replace the carrots with deseeded yellow peppers.

NUTRITIONAL VALUE PER SERVING

AS part of an intermittent diet plan, 1 serving provides your daily salty food 3 of your 5 daily vegetable portions. This meal provides 219 kcal per portion.

INGREDIENTS

- Calorie controlled cooking oil spray
- 1 medium onion, sliced
- 2 garlic cloves, thinly sliced
- 2 celery sticks, trimmed and thinly sliced
- 2 medium carrots or 2 yellow peppers, cut into 2cm/1in chunks
- 400g/14oz tin chopped tomatoes
- 1 vegetable stock cube
- 1 tsp dried mixed herbs
- 400g/14oz tin butter beans drained and rinsed
- 1 head young spring greens (approximately 125g/4½oz), trimmed and sliced

- sea salt and freshly ground black pepper

METHOD

1. Spray a large non-stick saucepan with oil and cook the onion, garlic, celery and carrots or peppers gently for 10 minutes, stirring regularly until softened.

2. Add 750ml/26fl oz water and the chopped tomatoes. Crumble over the stock cube and stir in the dried herbs. Bring to the boil, then reduce the heat to a simmer and cook for 20 minutes.

3. Season the soup with salt and pepper and add the spring greens and butterbeans. Return to a gentle simmer and cook for a further 3-4 minutes or until the greens are softened. Season to taste and serve in deep bowls.

Recipe Tips

Double the recipe if you fancy eating it over a couple of days. The butter beans can be substituted for other beans from your store cupboard if you don't have any.

LAMB AND FLAGEOLET BEAN STEW

Preparation time less than 30 minutes

Cooking time 1 to 2 hours

Serves Serves 4

This is a warming stew perfect for filling you up on a cold evening. Don't be put off by the long cooking time, this is an easy one-pot supper that will reward you for your patience.

NUTRITIONAL VALUE PER SERVING

As part of an intermittent diet plan, 1 serving provides, your daily salty food 3 of your 6 daily vegetable portions this meal provides 288 kcal per portion.

INGREDIENTS

- 1 tsp olive oil
- 350g/12oz lean lamb, cubed
- 16 pickling onions
- 1 garlic clove, crushed
- 600ml/20fl oz lamb stock (made with concentrated liquid stock)
- 200g can chopped tomatoes
- 1 bouquet garni
- 2 x 400g cans flageolet beans, drained and rinsed
- 320g/11oz green beans
- 250g/9oz cherry tomatoes
- freshly ground black pepper

METHOD

1. Heat the oil in a flameproof casserole or saucepan, add the lamb and fry for 3-4 minutes until browned all over. Remove the lamb from the casserole and set aside.

2. Add the onions and garlic to the pan and fry for 4-5 minutes, or until the onions are beginning to brown.

3. Return the lamb and any juices to the pan. Add the stock, tomatoes, bouquet garni and beans. Bring to the boil, stirring, then cover and simmer for 1 hour, or until the lamb is just tender.

4. Meanwhile, bring a pan of water to the boil and blanch the green beans. Place in bowl of ice-cold water.

5. Add the cherry tomatoes to the stew and season well with freshly ground black pepper. Continue to simmer for 10 minutes.

6. Divide the stew between four plates; place the green beans alongside and serve.

Recipe Tips
This dish could be made the night before and heated up.

CHILI AND CORIANDER FISH PARCEL

Preparation time 1-2 hours

Cooking time 10 to 30 minutes

Serves Serves 1

Baking fish is a great way to reduce calories. Give the fish extra oomph with chili and coriander.

NUTRITIONAL VALUE PER SERVING

For this recipe, you will need a blender or a food plan, 1 serving provides 1 of your 6 daily vegetable processor. As part of an intermittent diet portions and 148 calories.

INGREDIENTS

- 125g/4½oz cod, coaly or haddock fillet
- 2 tsp lemon juice
- 1 tbsp fresh coriander leaves
- 1 garlic clove, roughly chopped
- 1 green chili, deseeded and chopped
- ¼ tsp sugar
- 2 tbsp natural yoghurt
- 80g/3oz mange tout, steamed, to serve

METHOD

1. Preheat the oven to 200C/180C Fan/Gas 6.

2. Place the fish in a non-metallic dish and sprinkle with the lemon juice. Cover and leave in the fridge to marinate for 15-20 minutes.

3. Put the coriander, garlic and chili in a food processor or blender and process until the mixture forms a paste. Add the sugar and yoghurt and briefly process to blend.

4. Lay the fish on a sheet of foil. Coat the fish on both sides with the paste. Gather up the foil loosely and turn over at the top to seal. Return to the fridge for at least 1 hour.

5. Place the parcel on a baking tray and bake for about 15 minutes, or until the fish is just cooked. Serve with the mange tout.

STIR-FRIED PORK WITH GINGER AND SOY SAUCE

Preparation time less than 30 minutes

Cooking time 10 to 30 minutes

Serves Serves 2

This low calorie, stir-fried pork is quick and easy while still delivering on flavor, and helping you on your way to getting five a day.

NUTRITIONAL VALUE PER SERVING

As part of an intermittent diet plan, 1 serving provides your daily salty food 3 of your 5 daily vegetable portions, this meal provides 250 kcal per portion.

INGREDIENTS

- 250g/9oz pork tenderloin, all visible fat removed, cut into chunks
- 1 tsp cornflour
- 2 tbsp dark soy sauce
- low-calorie cooking spray
- 150g/5½oz button mushrooms, sliced
- 2 red peppers, deseeded and sliced
- 75g/2½oz mangetout, trimmed
- 15g/½oz fresh root ginger, cut into thin matchsticks
- 1 garlic clove, thinly sliced
- 4 spring onions, cut into short lengths
- freshly ground black pepper

METHOD

1. Season the pork with pepper. Mix the cornflour with two tablespoons of cold water until smooth, then stir in the soy sauce.

2. Spray a large wok, or deep frying pan, with cooking spray and place over a high heat. Stir-fry the pork for 1-2 minutes, or until lightly browned but not cooked through. Transfer to a plate.

3. Return the pan to the heat, reduce the heat a little and spray with more oil. Stir-fry the mushrooms and pepper for 2 minutes. Add the mange tout and cook for a minute. Add the ginger, garlic and spring onions and stir-fry for a few seconds.

4. Return the pork to the pan and pour over the soy sauce mixture. Cook for 1-2 minutes, or until the sauce has thickened and the pork is cooked through. Serve immediately.

HOW TO EAT ON FASTING DAYS...?

There is no rule for what or when to eat on fasting days. Some people function best by beginning the day with a small breakfast, while others find it best to start eating as late as possible. Generally, there are two meal patterns that people follow:

1. Three small meals: Usually breakfast, lunch and dinner.
2. Two slightly bigger meals: Only lunch and dinner.

Since calorie intake is limited 500 calories for women and 600 calories for men — it makes sense to use your calorie budget wisely.
Try to focus on nutritious, high-fibre, high-protein foods that will make you feel full without consuming too many calories.
Soups are a great option on fast days. Studies have shown that they may make you feel more full than the same ingredients in original form, or foods with the same calorie content. Here are a few examples of foods that may be suitable for fast days:

- A generous portion of vegetables
- Natural yogurt with berries
- Boiled or baked eggs.
- Grilled fish or lean meat
- Cauliflower rice
- Soups (for example miso, tomato, cauliflower or vegetable)
- Low-calorie cup soups
- Black coffee
- Tea
- Still or sparkling water

Given following chart will be helpful to get battcr benefits of 5:2 intermittent fasting one-month diet plan.

5:2 INTERMITTENT FASTING DAY BY DAY ONE MONTH DIET PLAN.

	Breakfast	Lunch	Dinner
Monday	Fast Day – 4 tasty and satisfying Fastpacks, 100% nutrition minus the calories		
Tuesday	Porridge with cinnamon, sliced apple and sultanas	Beetroot and walnut dip with mixed veg dippers	Walnut and anchovy crusted salmon
Wednesday	Nectarine, yoghurt and granola breakfast pot	Tomato and feta bruschetta	Roasted vegetables with pearl barley & balsamic dressing
Thursday	Fast Day – 4 tasty and satisfying Fastpacks, 100% nutrition minus the calories		
Friday	Asparagus and red pepper omelette	Salad niçoise	Chilli con carne
Saturday	Greek yoghurt with toasted almonds and berry compote	Baked sweet potato with a spring onion and crème fraiche topping	Caribbean chicken with fruity black bean sauce
Sunday	Scrambled egg on multigrain, multi-seeded bread with smoked salmon	Gazpacho	Rich pork casserole with mushrooms and soy sauce

In this plan, you fast only two days a wseek. You are allowed to eat during your fast days, but only a very small caloric intake

THE BOTTOM LINE

The 5:2 diet is an easy, effective way to lose weight and improve metabolic health. Many people find it much easier to stick to than a conventional calorie-restricted diet. If you're looking to lose weight or improve your health, the 5:2 diet is definitely something to consider.

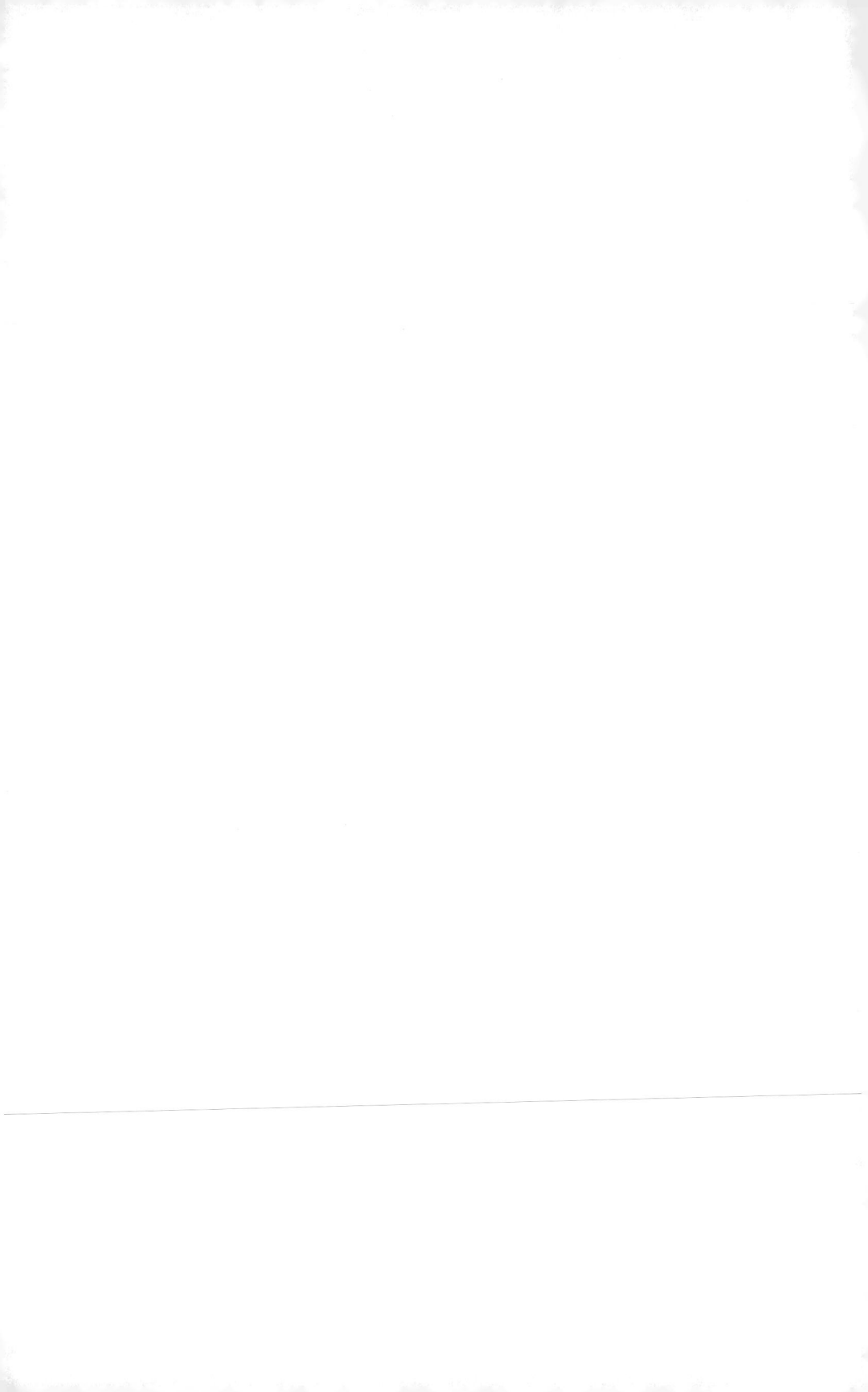

Made in the USA
Monee, IL
02 March 2020